Imperial Secrets *of* HEALTH · AND · LONGEVITY

D0939305

Imperial Secrets *of* HEALTH · AND · LONGEVITY

壽

BOB FLAWS

· BLUE POPPY PRESS ·

Published by:

BLUE POPPY PRESS, INC.
3450 Penrose Place, Suite 110
BOULDER, CO 80301

First Edition, January, 1994
Second Printing, May, 1998

ISBN 0-936185-51-1

COMP Designation: Original work

Printed at Johnson Printing in Boulder, CO, on acid free, elementally chlorine-free paper
Cover design by Bob Schram, Bookends Design

10 9 8 7 6 5 4 3 2

PREFACE

Back in the 1920s and 30s, a young Japanese acupuncturist was working in France. His name among Westerners was George Ohsawa. After treating Westerners for some time with acupuncture, he came to the conclusion that such treatment was merely a bandaid. He saw that as long as Westerners did not know how to live healthy lives, all his treatments were only stop-gap measures. As long as his patients did not eat right and live moderately, they either continued to be sick or got sick again soon after discontinuing treatment. He realized that he was treating people who were already ill and that the cause of their illness was, unlike in undeveloped countries, primarily the result of improper diet and lifestyle. Therefore, Ohsawa gave up the clinical practice of acupuncture and devoted the rest of his life to teaching Westerners how to live according to Oriental principles of longevity and good health. His teachings came to be known as Macrobiotics which is only a Greek way of saying big or long life.

As an American acupuncturist and doctor of Traditional Chinese Medicine, I too have come to the realization that, although acupuncture and Chinese herbal medicine are very effective remedially, the best thing I can do for Western patients is to make better known the traditional Chinese teachings on health preservation. The premier classic of Chinese medicine, the *Nei Jing (Inner Classic)*, says that treating disease after it arises is like beginning to dig a well after one has become thirsty or like forging spears after war has already broken out. It classifies this as the practice of inferior medicine. Likewise, the greatest Chinese doctor of the Tang dynasty, Sun Si-miao, said that the highest doctor is the teacher of the intentions of society. Further, Sun said that the good doctor first alters the patient's diet and lifestyle and only if that fails to effect a cure should they prescribe acupuncture and remedial herbal medicine. Sun Si-miao is also called the Immortal Sun since he lived to the age of 101, obviously practicing what he preached.

Frequently I take a walk on our outside mall in Boulder and former patients come up to me to say hello. It is not uncommon for them to begin by saying that they keep meaning to come in to see me in my clinic. It's almost as if they were apologizing. They then tell me that whenever their symptoms flare back up, they remember what I told them about their diet and lifestyle. If they follow that advice, their symptoms go away and then they don't need to come to get treatment from me. Far from making me unhappy, this is music to my ears. Whenever I hear this I am delighted, since this is my highest goal as a doctor of Chinese medicine. It means that I have taught them how to control their own health and wellbeing through their diet and lifestyle. Although I hope and intend to continue the clinical practice of acupuncture and Chinese herbal medicine for many more years, I also want to do everything possible to enlighten modern society to the age-old Oriental principles of health preservation and the nourishment of life. Thus I have written this book.

Bob Flaws
Boulder, CO

CONTENTS

Preface, v

Contents, vii

Introduction, 1

1
The Chinese Theory of Life & Death, 7

2
A Healthy, Regular Lifestyle, 13

3
Eating for Longevity, 21

4
Moderation in Sex, 41

5
Rest & Relaxation, 51

6
Dao Yin
Self-massage, 59

7
Exercise & Stretching, 69

8
Qi Gong, 77

9
Chinese Herbal Medicine, 87

10
Treating Illness Early, 95

11
Conclusion, 101

Index, 107

INTRODUCTION

People everywhere desire to live long, productive, happy, and healthy lives. In particular, the Chinese have traditionally made the search for longevity a conscious and integral part of their culture. Although all three major religions in China––Confucianism, Daoism, and Buddhism––include teachings on and practices for the attainment of long life, Chen Ying-ning, an early twentieth century Chinese authority on longevity practices, believed, in fact, that the study of immortality (*xian xue*) in China predates all three of these schools and constitutes a fourth school which, he said, is the most typically Chinese of all.[1] And, from a material point of view, who in China had more reason to live a long and healthy life than the emperors? As absolute monarchs, they had complete power, almost limitless wealth, and literally hundreds of concubines providing sex on demand. Theirs was a life of almost unimaginable luxury, and history records that most of the Chinese emperors were concerned with and, in some cases, preoccupied by the search for longevity, if not immortality.

However, the record also shows that few of these Chinese emperors lived into full old age. Most died young in their

---

1   Robert, Yves, "*Chen Yingning, Un Immortel dan le Siecle*", *Medécine Chinoise & Medécines Orientales*, No. 4, 1993, p. 52

thirties and forties, some even in their twenties. Some died because of ingesting so-called elixirs of immortality manufactured from toxic substances such as mercury. Thinking that a pill could make them immortal, they gullibly trusted their lives to quacks and poisoned themselves. Yet most of the Chinese emperors who died relatively young, and that was the majority, died because of their unregulated desires, indulgence in rich foods and wine, and lack of exercise. If one looks at the length of reigns from the Ming (1368-1644 AD) and Qing (1644-1911 AD) dynasties, we see that the average length of reign of the 27 emperors during this period lasted only a little over 19 years. If one assumes that most of these emperors ascended the throne in their teens and twenties, this means they died in the prime of their lives with seemingly everything to live for.

One notable exception to this trend was Qian Long, the fourth of the Manchu or Qing emperors. Qian Long reigned from 1736-1796 AD or a total of 60 years. He lived till well into his eighties. Why did Qian Long live so long when other emperors with the same material and medical resources at their command tended to die young? Qian Long left behind 14 secrets of longevity to which he credited his long life. These secrets were:

1. Rise early, find a place with pure fresh air, inhale deeply, and exhale the stale air
2. Use herbs and special foods to restore the *qi* (pronounced chee) or energy
3. Click the teeth together
4. Swallow the saliva
5. Massage the ears
6. Rub the nose
7. Roll the eyes

2

8. Knead the feet
9. Stretch the limbs
10. Raise the anus
11. Do not speak while eating
12. Do not chat when lying down
13. Do not drink to excess
14. Do not indulge in sex[2]

If one looks at this list of 14 secrets, one can divide these admonitions into several categories. First, Qian Long is advising people to get up early and not lay about in bed all day. In order to get up early, one also has to go to bed at a reasonable hour. Therefore, the first part of secret number one is to keep a regular life schedule. Secondly, Qian Long says to breathe deeply and exhale the stale air. Breathing exercises in China are called *qi gong*. *Qi* means energy and *gong* means to work or train. One's energy is intimately associated with one's breath and *qi gong* exercises are an integral part of Chinese longevity practices. Third, use herbs and foods to restore one's qi. This also has two parts. The first has to do with Chinese herbal medicine. There are special Chinese herbs which supplement one's *qi* or vitality and which nourish the various organs and body functions. In addition, proper diet is fundamental to attaining good health and long life.

Secrets three through 10 all have to do with getting regular exercise. However, beyond regular exercise such as stretching, Qian Long advises self-massaging specific body parts. As we will see below, each of the body parts mentioned is believed to represent the entire body and all its organs and thus massaging

_____

[2]   Chen Ke-ji, "From Emperors to Fisheyes, A Conversation about Chinese Medicine with Dr. Chen Keji", *Heaven Earth, The Chinese Art of Living*, May 1992, Vol. 2, No. 1, p. 7

these parts affects the entire organism inside and out, regulating and stimulating its functions.

Admonitions 11 and 12 have to do with only doing one thing at a time. When eating, just eat. When resting, just rest. I believe Qian Long is saying that one should not allow one's mind to race about attempting to do a million things at once. Further, Admonitions 11 and 12 both have to do with economy of speech. Admonition 13, not to drink to excess means not to overindulge in alcohol so as to avoid engendering dampness and heat. Number 14 counsels against indulging in sex, but it does not necessarily mean to forego sex altogether.

Taken as a whole, these 14 so-called secrets can be summed up as:

> A moderate and regular life schedule
> Proper diet
> Mental equipoise
> Adequate rest
> Regular exercise and especially stretching
> Self-massage
> *Qi gong* exercises
> Moderation in the drinking of alcohol
> Moderation in sex
> Use of Chinese herbal medicinals

In the following chapters we will look at the Chinese teachings concerning each of these topics. Qian Long was only one of numerous Chinese to leave behind their prescriptions for long life. In fact, in China, there is a voluminous literature on this subject. The material which follows is based on my research of this literature, on my experience as a doctor of

Traditional Chinese Medicine or TCM, and on my own personal experience as well. As a physician, I am certain that the practice of this ancient Chinese wisdom does result in increased health and wellbeing. It can contribute to the healing of those already ill and prevent disease in those who are currently seemingly healthy. An old Chinese proverb says, "Before 30, you cheat disease, but after 30, disease cheats you." The sooner one implements even some of the suggestions contained herein, the sooner one will see the results.

1.

THE CHINESE THEORY
OF LIFE & DEATH

Before one can make sense out of the specific Chinese teachings on the preservation of health and cultivation of life in the chapters that follow, it is necessary to understand something about the Chinese ideas of life and death. When one understands the traditional Chinese concepts of how life is empowered and sustained, then the particular teachings in the following chapters will seem much more reasonable. These Chinese theories have developed independent of modern Western science and medicine. Nonetheless, they form a coherent and logical whole which has stood the test of time in clinical practice over not less than a hundred generations.

Qi

Qi means influence or energy. It is the Chinese concept for the motivating force behind all movement and transformation in the world and in our bodies. Every metabolic change occurring in our bodies, every movement, every sensation, and every thought is empowered by and is an expression of the movement of *qi*. As long as we have *qi*, we are alive. When we run out of *qi* or fail to make sufficient new *qi* to get us through our daily lives, we die.

At the moment of conception, we are endowed with *qi* from our parents. It is this force which empowers our growth and

7

transformation in the womb. It also allows us to take our first breath. However, once we begin breathing and eating, we are constantly making new *qi*. When food enters the stomach, the spleen (or at least the Chinese idea of the spleen) distills the finest essence of the food and sends this up to the lungs. As the lungs breathe in, the finest essence of the air combines with the finest essence of the food to form *qi*. This *qi* is then sent out to the rest of the body to empower its growth, activity, and repair.

Jing Essence

At the moment of conception, we are also endowed with a very potent substance called *jing* or essence. This essence forms the initial material out of which our body forms. It also can be transformed into *qi*, and, in fact, as we go through life, every movement of *qi* in our bodies involves some consumption of this prenatally endowed *jing* essence. It is this *jing* essence which determines our individual make-up and constitution. Its quality and quantity are finite at the moment of conception. In a sense, this essence is the ultimate source of *qi* in our bodies since to make *qi*, some of this essence must be consumed. This prenatal *jing* is stored primarily in the Chinese idea of the kidneys. When it is used up, natural death occurs in the same way as a candle goes out when it has burned through all its wax.

Happily there is another kind of *jing* essence in the body. There is also what is called acquired or postnatal *jing*. This essence is manufactured from whatever surplus of *qi* exists at the end of the day when we enter deep sleep. As explained above, we are constantly manufacturing *qi* from the air we breathe and the food we eat. If, in a day, we manufacture more *qi* than we use in that day's activities and functions, this excess *qi* is converted into acquired essence during sleep. This acquired essence bolsters the prenatal essence and slows down its consumption. The body uses this acquired essence and does not have to use as much prenatal essence.

When we are young and healthy and if we have adequate food and rest, we make abundant *qi* each day, more than enough to result in a surplus which can be converted into acquired essence. However, as we age, our bodily organs do not function as well as before and we no longer manufacture as much *qi* as we did in our youth. Therefore, we begin use up more and more of our prenatal essence. Eventually it becomes exhausted completely and we die.

Shen Spirit

In the Chinese literature, there are three treasures or *san bao*. These are the *jing*, *qi*, and *shen* or spirit. This *shen* represents consciousness and our higher mental faculties. It is also associated with our vitality, the lustre of our skin, the sparkle in our eyes, and the harmony and steadiness of our thought as expressed by the tone and articulation of our voice. Li Dong-yuan, one of the four greatest doctors of the Jin/Yuan dynasties (1280-1368 AD), had this to say of the relationship between the *jing, qi,* and *shen*:

> *Qi* is the forefather of spirit and essence is the child of *qi*. (Thus) *qi* is the root of essence and spirit. Great is *qi*!

9

When *qi* accumulates, it produces essence. When essence accumulates, it renders spirit wholesome.[1]

This passage not only explains how generation of abundant *qi* can accumulate to become acquired essence, it also suggests that there is a direct relationship between the *shen* spirit and the *jing* essence. When the essence accumulates, the spirit is wholesome. This relationship helps explain from the Chinese point of view why our mental functions deteriorate with age.

The Kidneys

According to Chinese medical theory, the kidneys are the organ which store the lion's share of the essence, both acquired and prenatal. In fact, Chinese medicine sees the kidneys as the primary organ controlling growth, maturation, aging, and natural death. From the Chinese point of view, we are only as old as the amount of essence we have consumed. Another way of saying this is that we are only as old as our kidneys. In Chinese medicine, the ears, bones, genitalia and reproductive capacity, hair on the top of the head, teeth, mental clarity, and visual acuity are all related to kidney function and *jing* essence. Therefore, as we age, our hearing becomes impaired, our bones become brittle, our libido decreases and our ability to procreate becomes exhausted, we bald, our teeth fall out, our mind becomes unclear, and so does our vision.

---

[1]   Li Dong-yuan, *The Treatise on the Spleen & Stomach, A Translation of the Pi Wei Lun*, trans. by Yang Shou-zhong, Blue Poppy Press, Boulder, CO, 1993, p. 261

Based on the above ideas, it is no wonder that Chinese systems for the preservation of health and nourishment of life primarily involve the following objectives:

1. Maximizing *qi* production
2. Minimizing *qi* consumption
3. Maximizing *jing* production
4. Minimizing *jing* consumption
5. Maximizing the health of the kidneys

As we will see below, each of the topics and practices discussed below address one or more of these objectives. They are the overriding themes which provide the rationale for the various specific practices which make up the Chinese approach to the preservation of health and cultivation of long life.

2.

A HEALTHY, REGULAR LIFESTYLE

In Chinese, the conscious promotion of health and longevity is referred to primarily as either *yang sheng*, the cultivation or nourishment of life, or as *bao jian*, the preservation of one's strength (*i.e.*, health). It is also sometimes referred to as *yang xing*, cultivating or nourishing one's nature, *she sheng*, containing or absorbing life, and *dao sheng*, the path of life. Following Emperor Qian Long's lead, the first element in this study is the cultivation of a regular lifestyle. In Chinese, this is *qi ju you chang*, having normalcy in one's rising and dwelling. This begins with conforming with nature (*ze ying zi ran*). Literally this means following and responding to nature. Humans exist within nature, or the universe, and our life functions are controlled by and resonate with the greater forces of the world of which we are but a part. By consciously identifying, understanding, and working with these greater forces and cycles, one can go with the flow of things and thereby conserve energy which would otherwise be squandered by bucking the tide. Hua Tuo, one of the most famous of all Chinese doctors, who lived to be 97 and only died because he was executed by the tyrant Cao Cao, said this of the holistic relationship between the universe and humankind:

> Humanity is sustained by heaven above and supported by earth below, and (is) aided by yang and assisted by yin. When heaven and earth are in normal condition, the qi in

humans is harmonious; if heaven and earth are in abnormal condition, the qi in humans will be topsy-turvy.[1]

Following the Changes in the Four Seasons

According to the *Nei Jing (Inner Classic)*, "He who would nourish life surely follows (the changes of) the four seasons, adapts to cold and heat, harmonizes joy and anger, and dwells in calm."[2] This means that people should adjust their life schedule and activities to conform to the changes of the four seasons. Spring and summer are *yang* seasons. *Yang* means warmth, activity, upward and outward movement, and growth. Thus spring and summer are times of growth and greater activity. Fall and winter are *yin* seasons. *Yin* means cold, relative quiescence, and downward and inward movement. Therefore, fall and winter are times of rest, inward reflection, and storage and recuperation.[3]

In particular, the *Nei Jing* says to rise early in the spring and to take a leisurely walk. One should let their hair hang down (both literally and figuratively) and stay relaxed in all endeavors. They should avoid becoming angry or uptight. Thus their *yang qi* or *yang* energy will sprout and grow similar

---

[1]   Hua Tuo, *Master Hua's Classic of the Central Viscera, A Translation of Hua Tuo's Zhong Zang Jing*, trans. by Yang Shou-zhong, Blue Poppy Press, Boulder, CO, 1993, p. 3

[2]   *Nei Jing (Inner Classic)*, *Ling Shu (Spiritual Axis)*, Chapter 8, "Root of Spirit"

[3]   In terms of the human organism, yin refers to the body's substance and especially to body fluids, blood, and essence. Yang refers to the body's function and is responsible for movement, warmth, transformation, containment, and defense.

to the green shoots sprouting and budding in nature. In the summer, one should also rise early in the morning and take a sunbath. They should try to maintain a cheerful, expansive frame of mind. It is okay to work hard physically in the summer to the point of sweating since one is full of vigor in this season of abundance and maturation. In the fall, people should go to bed early and try to maintain a tranquil mind. In particular, they should try to avoid anxiety. Physical activity should begin to be curtailed somewhat during this season of harvest. In winter, the *Nei Jing* counsels to go to bed early and to get up later. One should avoid cold and seek warmth and not perspire too much. Winter is a time for introspection and relative rest.

These basic guidelines were written over 2,000 years ago when people did not have central heat, good housing, warm clothing, and abundant food. Some of these suggestions may not be as important today as they were when life was more precarious and people were exposed to the elements more. However, there is merit to the idea of living with the seasons and modifying one's activities to conform to the seasons.

Keeping Regular Hours

The *Nei Jing* says that the *yang qi* of the body begins to grow at sunrise. The *yang qi* becomes exuberant at midday when the sun is brightest, and the *yang qi* begins to decrease at sunset. This daily growth and decline of *yang qi* suggests that humans should likewise rise at sunup, work during the middle of the day, and rest at sundown, remembering that *yang qi* is associated with function and activity. Further, Chinese medical theory says that the *qi* and blood of the body flow through certain channels or so-called meridians at certain times of the day in a rhythmic and orderly manner. These channels

15

connect with the internal organs and their function reflects the rhythmic ebb and flow of *qi* and blood over these channels. Thus the majority of humans are healthiest when they live a regular lifestyle, rising in the morning, working during the day, and sleeping at night. In addition, it is best to eat at the same times each day and establish a routine. This leads to harmony within the body and the smooth functioning of the internal organs. As Sun Guang-ren *et al.* say in *Health Preservation and Rehabilitation*:

> To keep regular hours, man should, first of all, work out a time schedule that tallies with the actual conditions of his constitution, surroundings and work. In the time schedule, a day's time should be reasonably allocated to labor or work, sports activities, recreational activities, meals, rest and sleep. Man should take the time schedule as a rule and act upon it perseveringly so as to foster good living habits. This is of important significance to preserving health and preventing disease, just as Sun Si-miao of the Tang dynasty said: "Those who are good at health preservation vary their time of rising and going to bed in accordance with the supersession of the seasons and keep regular hours in daily life."[4]

Several years ago, I had a patient who was in his late twenties. Because he could earn more money, he worked the graveyard shift from 12-8 AM. He suffered from chronic low back pain and tinnitus or ringing in his ears. These are symptoms of kidney weakness in Chinese medicine. I told him that I thought his late night work schedule was part of the problem.

---

[4]   Sun Guang-ren, Liu Zhao-cun, Li Hong-bo, Yang Si-qin, Chong Gui-qin, *Health Preservation and Rehabilitation*, ed. by Zhang En-qin, trans. by Li Xue-zhen *et al.*, Shanghai College of Traditional Chinese Medicine Press, Shanghai, 1990, p. 159-160

He then told me that at the plant at which he worked they had an employee clinic. This clinic performed wellness check-ups on all the workers and part of this wellness checkup included an assessment of one's biological age. One's chronological age is figured on the calendar from the day of birth. Everyone born on Feb. 20, 1946 will turn 50 on Feb. 20, 1996. Biological age, however, is the age the body is in terms of wear and tear. One 50-year-old might biologically be only 40 and another be biologically 60. This man was chronologically in his late twenties but biologically tested in his mid-thirties. He also told me that such advances in biological age were the norm in the workers on his shift. Kidney supplement herbs helped this man's symptoms, but they never completely disappeared since he was not willing to give up the graveyard shift.

Healthy Surroundings

Because people are not separate from but are an integral part of their environment, a person's surroundings greatly impact on one's health and wellbeing. In China, a science developed which was designed to diagnose the energy and influences on humans of any environment or building. This science is called *feng shui* or wind and water. Based on this art, one can pick places most conducive to one's health and success as well as alter their surroundings in a conscious and deliberate way, hence improving their health and chances of success. In the Chinese literature on the cultivation or nourishment of life, this topic is called *shi yi huan jing*, suitable or comfortable surroundings. Although the art of *feng shui* vis á vis health and longevity deserves a book of its own, there are a few principles which can be stated simply and succinctly.

17

First, according to the theory of health preservation of TCM, peaceful and secluded surroundings promote human health in both body and mind and help prolong life. Chinese experts on cultivation of life throughout the ages have consistently recommended living in peaceful secluded places with plenty of fresh air, sunshine, good ventilation, moderate humidity, and a minimum of pollution, noise, and hustle and bustle. Such places include the seashore, the countryside, and the mountains. It is said that one should live far enough away from a town so as not to be bothered by noise and unnecessary interruptions but not so far away as to make one's daily life difficult or onerous.

Secondly, since most people spend approximately half their lives within their house, the location and shape of that house is extremely important. Basically, *feng shui* masters are unanimous in recommending that one's house face south with the bedrooms on the east. Thus the front of the house receives the warmth of the sun throughout the day and the bedrooms receive the first rays of the sun waking and warming the residents early in the morning. In that way their *yang qi* can respond to the rising *yang* in the external environment. In addition, the house should be situated in a place where there is good soil and pure water surrounded by trees and flowers. If one lives in the city, one can at least try to have a pond and garden within sight of the house. These recommendations not only affect one's mood but also help insure proper lighting, warmth, and fresh air.

Lastly, one's bedroom is an especially important room in terms of one's health and longevity. People spend as much as a third of their lives in this room. A sound, restful, undisturbed sleep is vital to replenishing one's energy each day. Nothing takes its toll on one's energy any faster than failing to achieve

18

deep, restful sleep. Further, since during sleep all one's defenses are down, one is particularly vulnerable to the effects of any noxious or harmful energy. Such harmful energy can come from proximity to electrical appliances, including electric blankets and clocks, from subterranean water running under the bed, and from so-called *sha* or killing *qi* from a wrongly positioned bed. Chen Zhi, a Song dynasty (960-1280 AD) longevity expert, has also written that, "Bedrooms must be kept clean and tasteful, open and empty in summer and warm and tight in winter."[5]

As mentioned above, *feng shui* is its own art and science, and there is much more to know about *feng shui* and long life. For more information on particulars concerning location, architecture, and decorating and health, interested readers should see *Feng Shui, The Chinese Art of Placement* and *Interior Design with Feng Shui*.[6] However, it should be remembered that, as he felt the advance of age, the famous Dr. Sun Si-miao, the so-called Immortal Sun, moved to a secluded place with green hills and pure water where he built his house and ponds, planted trees and flowers, and died at 101 years of age.

---

[5] Chen Zhi, *Shou Qin Yang Nian Xin Shu (A New Book for Cultivating Long Life in [One's] Parents)*, quoted by Sun Guang-ren *et al.*, *op. cit.*, p. 156

[6] Rossbach, Sarah, *Feng Shui, The Chinese Art of Placement*, E.P. Dutton, Inc., NY, 1983; Rossbach, Sarah, *Interior Design with Feng Shui*, E.P. Dutton, Inc., NY, 1987

3.

EATING FOR LONGEVITY

In Chapter 1, we said that *qi* is made in part from the finest essence of the food we eat. Therefore proper diet is one of the most important facets of health preservation and the cultivation of life. Especially in rich and developed countries, improper diet is a major cause of disease and mortality. As a doctor, I have seen more than one patient literally kill themselves by eating improperly.

To understand the Chinese teachings on healthy eating we must begin with an analogy. Chinese doctors see the process of digestion as essentially a process of distillation. The stomach is likened to a fermentation vat. Food and liquids enter this vat to "rotten and ripen". Then the spleen, which is like the fire under the pot, provides the energy to separate off the finest essence from the food and liquids in the stomach. This finest essence (*jing wei*) is likened to a mist rising to the lungs similar to alcohol rising and condensing in a still. In terms of digestion, this finest essence is referred to as the clear (*qing*) part of the food and liquids ingested and this clear *qi* should rise upward. The dregs of the process of digestion are referred to as the turbid (*zhuo*) and this turbidity should descend to be excreted from the large intestine and urinary bladder. Thus the process of digestion can be spoken of as the separation of clear and turbid or the ascension of the clear and descension of the turbid. Further, the Chinese believe that this entire process is a warm transformation requiring adequate heat.

Clear, Light Food

Clear (*qing*), light or bland (*dan*) food is believed in China to be the healthiest. A *qing dan* diet consists primarily of vegetarian foods. This means grains, vegetables, and some fruits. In China, the word for food is often *gu* or grain. For instance, the *qi* manufactured from food is simply referred to as *gu* or grain *qi*. Along with grains, one should eat beans and bean products, such as tofu, which is highly nutritious as well as being easy to digest. There should be plenty of dark, leafy greens in the diet as well as red and yellow vegetables, such as beets, carrots, and squash. This follows the advise found in Chapter 22 of the *Su Wen (Simple Questions)*, "The five grains nourish; the five fruits assist; the five meats boost; and the five vegetables fill." Sun Si-miao advocated eating more "grains, beans, vegetables, and fruits whose flavors are naturally light and harmonious.[1] Likewise he said "Vegetables are indispensable at every meal."[2]

Although most Chinese authorities on the cultivation of life recommend a mostly vegetarian diet, they do not eschew all animal products. Sun Si-miao also recommended, "Eat those

---

[1] Sun Si-miao, quoted by Sun Guang-ren *et al.*, *Health Preservation and Rehabilitation*, Shanghai College of Traditional Chinese Medicine Press, Shanghai, 1988, p. 82, translated by the author

[2] *Ibid.*, p. 82

fish, meat, and fruit which boost people's (health)."[3] Thus, a small amount of meat, eggs, and dairy are recommended by most Chinese doctors. These foods are high in nutrition and are necessary in small amounts to rebuild and repair the body. However, they also tend to be hard to digest and can easily clog the system with unnecessary turbidity and phlegm. When animal protein is included in the diet, it should only be used as a flavoring and condiment or side dish, not the main course. When patients ask me how much meat to include in their diet, I typically counsel not more than 4 ounces of meat 3-4 times a week. Although Sun suggested that animal protein should be eaten, he also said, "The cuisine should not be sumptuous in fish and meat and is better to be kept thrifty and simple."[4] Similarly, Li Dong-yuan was unequivocal when he said, "One should eat more grains and less meat."[5]

Oils and fat as well as hot, pungent spices are the opposite of a *qing dan* diet. Li Dong-yuan, in his *Pi Wei Lun (Treatise on the Spleen & Stomach)*, states that spicy, hot foods injure and damage the original *qi*.[6] This original *qi* is the *qi* made from the food which becomes the basis for all the other *qi* in the body. Li Chan of the Ming dynasty, in his *Yi Xue Ru Men*

---

[3]   Sun Si-miao, quoted by Sun Guang-ren *et al.*, *Health Preservation and Rehabilitation*, Shanghai College of Traditional Chinese Medicine Press, Shanghai, 1988, p. 86

[4]   *Ibid.*, p. 14

[5]   *Ibid.*, p. 16

[6]   Li Dong-yuan, *Li Dong-yuan's Treatise on the Spleen and Stomach: A Translation of the Pi Wei Lun*, translated by Yang Shou-zhong, Blue Poppy Press, Boulder, CO, 1993, p. 62

(Entering the Gate of Medicine), says that one should also avoid fried, roasted, toasted, fermented, pickled in soy sauce, or hot natured foods since these dry the blood.[7] In sum, Ge Hong of the Eastern Jin dynasty said that a clear, light diet nourishes the stomach and eating less in general relieves the intestines.[8]

Zhu Dan-xi was one of the four great masters of medicine of the Jin-Yuan dynasties (1280-1368 AD). In his *Ge Zhi Yu Lun (Extra Treatises Based on Investigation & Inquiry)*, Master Zhu devotes an entire chapter to eating a *qing dan* or clear, bland diet. In his "Treatise on Eating Bland Food", he begins with the question:

> Some may ask, "The *Nei Jing (Inner Classic)* states that insufficient essence should be supplemented with flavors. It is also stated that the earth feeds human beings with the five flavors. The ancients began eating meat at the age of 50, but your honor, now as old as 70, (even yet) abstains completely from salt and vinegar. Have you acquired the *dao* (*i.e.*, achieved sainthood)? (If not,) how does your honor manage to keep your spirit thriving and your complexion shining?"

> The answer is that some of the flavors are a gift from heaven and others are produced by human endeavor. The gifts from heaven include, for instance, grains, beans, greens, and fruits which are moderate and harmonious flavors. when eaten as food for humans, these result in supplementing yin. These are what is referred to as flavor

---

[7]   Li Chan, *Yi Xue Ru Men (Entering the Gate of Medicine)*, quoted by Sun Guang-ren *et al.*, *op. cit.*, p. 84

[8]   Ge Hong, *Bao Pu Zi Nei Pian (Bao Pu-zi's Inner Treatises)*, quoted by Sun Guang-ren *et al.*, *op. cit.*, p. 86

in the *Nei Jing*. Those which human endeavor produces are the partially thick flavors made by means of brewing and blending in the process of cooking. These carry toxins that cause illness and fell life. It is these sort of flavors of which you are suspicious.[9]

According to Master Zhu, rice and other grains, beans, vegetables, and fruits are flavorful in and of themselves, and it is these sort of natural flavors which should form the basis of the healthy human diet. Whereas, artificially strong flavors created by fermentation and other such processes tend to include toxins which are harmful and cause disease. Zhu Dan-xi goes on to say:

People must eat whenever they are hungry. The virtue of earth is embodied in the sweetness and blandness of rice. Rice is a substance ascribed to yin and is most supplementing, but it should be taken with vegetables. The reason why it should go together with vegetables in order to replenish is the fear that (otherwise) it would cause detriment to the stomach if eaten in quantities... Vegetables are taken to assist rice in replenishing and fulfilling because they are able to course and free (the stomach) and make transformation (*i.e.*, digestion) easy.[10]

This paragraph implies that although, rice is the best grain for supplementing the human body, it should be eaten with sufficient vegetables. Rice, because it is "replenishing and fulfilling" is still somewhat heavy and can clog the digestive track if

---

[9] Zhu Dan-xi, *Ge Zhi Yu Lun (Extra Treatises Based on Investigation & Inquiry)*, "Treatise on Eating Bland Food", translated by Yang Shou-zhong, Blue Poppy Press, Boulder, CO, to be published in 1994

[10] *Ibid.*

eaten too much. Vegetables, on the other hand, are light and easily digestible. Eating sufficient vegetables with grains such as rice thus keeps the digestive track open and clear at the same time as the body is nourished and replenished.

Interestingly, the United States Department of Agriculture has recently released revised guidelines on healthy eating. Instead of the four food groups promulgated for so many years, the USDA is now using food pyramid to teach people the principles of a healthy diet. This pyramid shows grains and beans as the staple foods of the diet. Next in order of amount and importance come fruits and vegetables. Then come animal proteins in lesser amounts, with sugars, sweets, oils, and fats to be used only sparingly or on an occasional basis. This is essentially the Chinese idea of a *qing dan* diet.

Raw vs. Cooked Food

From the Chinese point of view, cooking food is nothing other than predigesting it since all food once it is eaten must be turned into 100°F soup in the stomach. For thousands of years, Chinese have believed that the majority of food should be eaten cooked as opposed to raw. However, this does not mean that food should be overcooked. On the contrary, food should be freshly prepared and only lightly steamed or boiled. This light cooking makes digestion easier and the nutrients in foods more easily assimilable. In addition, cooking foods generally releases their flavor and aroma, thus stimulating the appetite. As one ages or if one is chronically ill, the appetite may become depressed. Therefore, lightly cooking foods helps maintain a healthy appetite in order that adequate *qi* may be created.

In particular, it is important to cook otherwise hard to digest foods, such as grains. Grains should first be washed and then cooked until soft to the teeth. They should not be hard or crunchy. The older or weaker a person is, the more thoroughly grains should be cooked. This is in inverse proportion to the power of digestion. As a child, I remember my mother and grandmother making me soups and broths when I was ill to help me recuperate. This makes perfect sense from the Chinese perspective. In China, a favorite food for the young, the ill, or the aged is *shi fan* or water rice. This is made by cooking rice in several more times water than usual and typically overnight. This results in a thin rice soup. Then vegetables, eggs, fish, or Chinese herbs can be par-boiled in this soup just prior to serving as an especially easy to digest but nutritious food. Noodles are, likewise, an easily digested form of grains.

Li Dong-yuan, mentioned above, believed it was important not to eat or drink excessively cold foods and liquids. Since the process of digestion is a process of making 100°F soup, eating chilled or frozen foods or drinking iced water or drinks can douse the fire of digestion. According to Li, in that case, clear and turbid are not separated and the result is turbid dampness and phlegm which obstructs the free flow of *qi* and blood. This then can give rise to a large number of diseases. In fact, Sun Bing-yan, a famous contemporary Chinese cancer specialist, believes that such cold and damp turbidity is at the root of most cancers.[11] This is especially interesting since some Western cancer theorists believe that cancer patients lack adequate digestive enzymes.

---

[11] Sun Bing-yan, *Cancer Treatment and Prevention with Traditional Chinese Medicine*, Offete Enterprises, Inc., San Mateo, CA, 1991, p. 61

Many years ago when I was studying with a chiropractor, he told a story about Dr. Speer. Dr. Speer was a chiropractor who built a chiropractic hospital in Denver. He became interested in the causes of longevity and did a survey of centenarians. When he asked them what was the secret of their long life, he got back many contradictory answers. Some said they smoked and some said they never smoked. Some said they drank and others said they were teetotallers. Some ate meat and some were vegetarians. The one common thread, however, was that none of them ate anything either excessively cold or excessively hot.

Eating the Right Amount

Failure to either eat when hungry or drink when thirsty results in exhaustion of the source of *qi* and blood. On the other hand, excess food injures the spleen and stomach, impairing digestion. TCM describes five results from overeating. These include too frequent defecation, too frequent urination, disturbed sleep, obesity, and indigestion. Most TCM practitioners throughout history have suggested that one should stop eating when one is 70% full. This allows room for good and thorough digestion to take place.

Set Time, Set Amount

Practitioners of TCM believe that eating at regular, fixed times each day is best. This is because the body functions according to circadian rhythms which are repeated daily as discussed above. Therefore, it is said that having meals at fixed times can keep the body free from suffering. Basically, one should eat like a prince at breakfast, like a merchant at lunch, and like a pauper at dinner. This means that one's meals should become smaller as the day progresses and that one should not eat before bed. This is so the body has a chance to completely digest the day's food before going to sleep so that the food does not ferment in the intestines unhealthily.

The power of digestion in the elderly or the ill is usually decreased or impaired. For this reason, those who are aged or are sick are advised to eat smaller meals more often throughout the day. This allows the stomach and intestines the opportunity to digest food more easily and thus keep one's *qi* healthy and abundant.

However, even though one is advised to eat at fixed times each day, one should not eat if they are emotionally upset. If one eats when upset, because the ascent and descent of *qi* is disordered at that time, the pure will not be separated from the turbid and food stagnation is likely to occur. In that case, it is better to eat later than usual after one has calmed down rather than eating on schedule when one is upset.

Good Dining Practices

Besides eating only a moderate amount, there are several other points Chinese longevity specialists make *vis á vis* the process of eating. First, one should take their time. As Yuan Li-ren and Liu Xiao-ming say:

> It is important to eat slowly, chew thoroughly before swallowing, and never to "wolf down" food. Eating hurriedly results in indigestion. Eating too much at one meal quickly overburdens the gastrointestinal tract and may

29

lead to accidents like choking, irritation and coughing that injure the body.[12]

The process of turning food into 100°F soup begins with chewing in the mouth. The teeth puree the food so that it may be digested in the stomach. It is very important to take time and chew one's food thoroughly and to eat slowly.

Secondly, one should concentrate on dining. One should try not to be distracted by their thoughts while eating. As Qian Long advised, one should not chatter away while eating. If one is disturbed by distracting thoughts during a meal and eats absentmindedly, one's appetite will inevitably be affected, resulting in poor digestion and assimilation.

Third, one should rub their abdomen after meals. This can markedly improve digestion and absorption of nutrients. It is simple to do but can have profound effect. First, rub one's hands together till they are warm. Then place them on the abdomen and rub in large circles from right to left 20-30 times. Pause and then reverse these circles, rubbing from left to right 20-30 times. People with poor digestion or who are overweight should increase the number of repetitions up to 2-300 times. If one has a tendency to constipation, one should rub only right to left, following the course of the large intestine.

And finally, one should take a short walk after meals to also aid the digestion. In the nineteenth century in the West, this was referred to as a postprandial constitutional. After a short rest, one should take a leisurely stroll in order to mildly

---

[12]   Yuan Li-ren & Liu Xiao-ming, "Traditional Chinese Methods of Health Preservation", *The Journal of Chinese Medicine*, UK, No. 41, Jan. 1993, p. 37

stimulate their flow of *qi* and blood. This helps the clear to rise and the turbid to descend. In China there is a saying, "Walk 100 paces after meals and one can live 99 years."

Harmonizing the Five Flavors

Chapter 63 of the *Ling Shu (Spiritual Pivot; i.e.,* the second part of the *Nei Jing)* says that only a diet comprised of all five flavors—sweet, bitter, acrid, sour, and salty—can keep the bones straight, the sinews supple, the *qi* and blood flowing, the pores closed, and the functioning of the five major organs coordinated and balanced harmoniously. Conversely, persistent addiction to a certain flavor will lead to its accumulation within the body and , in the course of time, will result in loss of balance of the organs and bowels.

Chapter 3 of the *Su Wen (Simple Questions; i.e.,* the first part of the *Nei Jing)* says that too much sour causes liver *qi* repletion or fullness with consequent spleen *qi* exhaustion. Too much salt taxes the *qi* of the large bones and withers the flesh in addition to repressing heart *qi*. Too much sweet causes heart *qi* to be full and stuffy, the facial color blackish, and the kidney *qi* not balanced. Too much bitter causes the spleen *qi* to lose its moisture and the stomach *qi* to become too broad and distended. Too much acrid or pungent causes the sinews to be slack and the vessels stopped up, while the essence and spirit suffer disaster.

Harmonizing Hot & Cold

In addition, guarding against partialities in food also means balancing foods of both hot and cold natures. Besides the five flavors, each food has its own nature. This refers to its inherent temperature and that temperature's effect on the

31

body. As mentioned above, too much hot food injures the original *qi* and body fluids or *yin*. While too much cold injures the spleen and stomach *qi* and damages the digestive ability.

Choosing Food Based on Constitutional Type

Each person has a particular constitution. This constitution predisposes one towards certain types of problems and diseases. Different schools within Chinese medicine have historically used different systems for classifying various constitutional types. In modern TCM, we can divide most people into one of four categories. These are the wood/fire type, the phlegm/damp type, the yin vacuity type, and the yang vacuity type.

The wood/fire type is mesomorphic, meaning that they are moderately built. They are muscular and tight, possibly stringy, angular, strong willed, and possibly aggressive or nervous. Many people during their twenties, thirties, and even forties belong to this wood/fire type. Fire or heat in such persons is excessive or at least potentially excessive and this fire can, if it gets out of control, damage and consume the *qi*. Wood/fire types should eat more moistening foods, such as fruits and vegetables, millet, beans, and eggs. On the other hand, they should avoid hot foods, such as beef and lamb.

Phlegm/damp persons tend to be obese or endomorphic. Their flesh is typically atonic. According to TCM theory, accumulation of phlegm and dampness is primarily due to weak spleen and stomach function. therefore, in order to benefit digestion, more light, easily digestible food, such as cooked vegetables, is recommended along with bland tasting foods which seep dampness from the body by promoting urination. such persons should stay away from or minimize foods which tend to generate more body fluids, such as greasy, fatty foods, milk and milk products.

Yin vacuity (empty or deficient) persons mostly refer to people who have entered middle age. In addition, ectomorphic or very thin, nervous people may be constitutionally yin vacuitous from birth. It is said in Chinese, *nian si shi, yin qi si ban*. This means that by 40 years of age, the healthy *yin qi* is automatically reduced by half, since the process of life itself is the consumption and transformation of *yin* substance by *yang qi* or activity or function. People with a yin vacuity constitution, whether from birth or due to aging, should eat light foods which nourish *yin* by being easy to digest and thus being easily transformed into *qi* and blood.If there is abundant *qi* and blood, it will as described above, be transformed into *jing* essence at night during sleep. This *jing* is the root of healthy *yin* substance in the body. such light, easy to digest but nonetheless *yin*-nourishing foods include fruits, vegetables, milk, eggs, and bean products, such as tofu.

Yang vacuity (empty or deficient) persons mostly refer to the truly aged. As one enters the last decades of life, the fire at the gate of life begins to decline and with this one's metabolism slows and their body warmth decreases. It is also possible for a person to be born with a constitutional insufficiency of *yang qi*. People who are *yang* vacuitous should eat more acrid, warm foods, such as fish, fowl, beef, lamb, ginger, and pepper. They should be careful, on the other hand, to avoid cold, raw, or uncooked foods, cold drinks, and most fruits.

Balancing Food in the Four Seasons

One of the strong points of TCM theory is its insistence that true health can only be attained when the internal microcosm

33

is in harmonious balance with the external macrocosm. Thus TCM practitioners have long taught that one must use different acupuncture points, different herbs, and different foods during the different seasons in order for the part, the individual, to remain in balance with the whole, the external cosmos.

Therefore, during spring, it is advised that one eat more sweet than sour food so as to nourish the spleen. This is based on the ancient Chinese five phase theory correlating each phase with a season of the year, organ in the body, a flavor, color, musical note, number, etc. In addition, one should not overeat. This is based on the fact that the liver is associated with spring and rules free and unobstructed coursing and discharge of the *qi* and blood. If one overeats, this will block the free flow of *qi* and thus can harm the liver.

In the summer, the heart is replete and the kidneys are vacuous (empty). Therefore, one should eat light, easily digestible food and shun greasy, tough, hard to digest food which might aggravate fire and heat within the body. Rather one should eat nutritious fruits and vegetables. One may partake of drinks that are by nature cold, such as mung bean soup, but should not overindulge in physically cold, chilled, or iced drinks which can easily injure the spleen and stomach and damage the kidneys.

In the fall, one should continue avoiding overdrinking cold drinks and eating too many raw, cold foods. Because the weather is hot and dry during this season (early August to early November), one may feel thirsty and parched. However, indulging and assuaging this thirst with chilled drinks and frozen treats only damages the spleen and stomach *yang qi*. To help allay this thirst, one may eat apples and pears.

Winter is a time of storage and repair. Thus this is a time when supplementing, highly nutritious food can and should be taken. Such supplementing foods according to TCM theory include beef, lamb, chicken, and duck. In addition, TCM practitioners have traditionally felt that drinking a little alcohol during winter is beneficial.

Besides seasonal changes, foods should be chosen according to differences in local conditions. More warm, hot foods should be eaten in cold climes. More cold or cool foods should be eaten in hot areas. More acrid, spicy foods should be eaten in damp locations. More sweet, moistening foods should be eaten in dry environments.

Moderation in the Consumption of Liquids

Qian Long's thirteenth piece of advice for those seeking to live a long and healthy life is not to drink to excess. In the West, many people think drinking more liquids every day is good for one's health. Certainly, it is important to drink enough liquids. However, the body is not a sieve. Liquids consumed must pass through the digestive system and must be actively processed by the body's qi mechanism.

According to Chinese medical theory, the three organs which control water metabolism in the body are the lungs, spleen, and kidneys. Of these three, the spleen and kidneys are the most important. The spleen controls the movement and transformation of all liquids in the body. Liquids are a yin substance. They are moved and transformed by yang qi. If one drinks too many liquids in general, but cold liquids or excessive liquids with meals in particular, spleen qi will not be able to transform and transport these properly. In this case, these liquids will accumulate and back up, transforming into

35

phlegm and pathological dampness. This phlegm and dampness will then obstruct the free and open flow of qi and blood leading to stagnation and stasis. In addition, the spleen qi will become weak in trying to deal with this excess of fluids. Since the spleen is the root of qi and blood production, qi and blood will also not be adequately generated and transformed, eventually leading to an insufficiency of acquired essence.

The kidneys, on the other hand, primarily govern the excretion of fluids sent down to them by the downbearing qi of the lungs. If one drinks too many liquids, the kidney qi will become overburdened by having to excrete these excess fluids as urine. According to Chinese medical theory, urine does not flow from the body like water in a stream, but is moved or pushed out of the body by kidney qi. Therefore, over time, drinking excessive liquids results in exhausting and consuming kidney qi unnecessarily and prematurely. Since the kidneys are the so-called prenatal root and repository of the body's essence, kidney qi vacuity has a direct impact on the acceleration of the aging process.

Since all food must be turned into 100°F soup in the stomach for digestion and absorption to take place, it is very helpful to drink a cup of hot liquid, such as green tea or herbal tea with meals. It is deleterious however to drink excessive liquids with meals, or any cold liquids with meals. Otherwise, one should drink when thirsty between meals.

When my uncle was a college student, he developed stomach pain. He went to a doctor who was considered quite radical in his day. He put my uncle on a special diet, part of which was not drinking liquids with meals and not eating sugary deserts with meals. My uncle followed this diet for more than 60 years. Till his death in his late 80's, he always looked and behaved like a man 20 years younger than he was.

Moderation in the Use of Alcohol

Jin Zi-jiu was a late nineteenth century Chinese doctor living in Hangzhou, south of Shanghai. He left behind a book entitled *Jin Zi Jiu Zhuan Ji (Jin Zi-jiu's Collected Writings)*. In that book, Dr. Jin describes the nature and effects of alcohol from a Chinese medical perspective. His description reads:

> Alcohol has a volatile nature that damages the spirit and injures the blood. Its energy is hot and it leads to wasting and decline (of qi and yin). Alcohol first enters the gallbladder and liver where gallbladder fire explodes. The qi loses its restraint and descension. Liver yin (*i.e.*, the blood) is looted. The blood becomes unsettled and, as a result, counterflow ascension with vomiting of blood can occur. Moreover, alcohol is damp as well as hot. Dampness damages the spleen. This creates stagnant food and phlegm which easily gum the (qi) mechanism.[13]

Thus it is easy to see even of one is not an expert in Chinese medical theory that drinking too much alcohol is harmful to one's health. However, alcohol's hot, acrid nature does also have some benefits when drunk in moderation. It quickens the flow of qi and blood and thus aids the circulation. Chinese doctors believe that a little alcohol drunk regularly and especially during the winter is good for one. The issue is one entirely of moderation.

---

[13] Jin Zi-jiu, *Jin Zi Jiu Zhuan Ji (Jin Zi-jiu's Collected Writings)*, People's Health Publishing Society, Beijing, 1982, p.35-6

Remedial Dietary Therapy

The foregoing principles are general guidelines for longterm health maintenance. Whenever a person becomes ill, they should modify their diet on the basis of a professional Chinese diagnosis. During an acute or active disease, it is important that the patient follow the doctor's advise about what to eat and not to eat. Only if they do can they expect the best results from other therapies such as acupuncture and Chinese herbal medicine. In Chinese medicine, there are specific dietary regimens and foods for people with hypertension, high cholesterol, cancer, arthritis, irritable bowel syndrome, and other such diseases. Nevertheless, the *qing dan* diet is the foundation of Chinese dietary therapy even in such cases requiring remedial treatment.

The above is only a condensed summary of Chinese dietary wisdom as it pertains to the maintenance of good health and the cultivation of long life. For descriptions of the tastes, temperatures, and medicinal effects of individual foods, the reader is advised to see *Prince Wen Hui's Cook: Chinese Dietary Therapy*.[14] Readers are also referred to my *Arisal of the Clear: A Simple Guide to Healthy Eating According to Traditional Chinese Medicine*[15] for more detailed information on Chinese dietary principles and health. This book answers many questions Westerners typically have and addresses many

---

[14] Flaws, Bob & Wolfe, Honora Lee, *Prince Wen Hui's Cook: Chinese Dietary Therapy*, Paradigm Publications, Brookline, MA, 1983

[15] Flaws, Bob, *Arisal of the Clear: A Simple Guide to Healthy Eating According to Traditional Chinese Medicine*, Blue Poppy Press, Boulder, CO, 1991

modern issues concerning diet, such as food allergies, cholesterol, and candidiasis.

Thirteen hundred years ago, Sun Si-miao said, "Those who are ignorant about food cannot survive."[16] As a Chinese doctor in clinical practice in the West, I find faulty diet to be one of, if not the most, common causes of disease among my patients. The more of the above dietary wisdom a person can put into practice, the healthier they will be.

---

[16]   Quoted by Sun, James, "Pillars of Longevity", *Qigong, Health & Healing for the 21st Century*, Winter 1993, p. 20

4.

MODERATION IN SEX

In the *Lao Lao Heng Yan (Perennial Sayings in Gerontology)*, it is said, "The sexual desire of men and women is like the *dao* of *yin* and *yang* in nature."[1] This means that sexual desire in men and women is perfectly natural and of itself neither good nor bad. According to Chinese medical theory, either too much or too little sex can be harmful to the health. Ge Hong (281-341 AD), a famous Jin dynasty doctor and Daoist adept, summed this up nicely in his *Nei Pian (Inner Writings)*:

> It is not all right for humans to sever their sexual desire.
> *Yin* and *yang* (can then) not communicate. This will lead to
> diseases due to accumulation and stagnation. Those who
> suffer from diseases due to bitterness hidden in their mind
> (in turn) due to protracted suppression of their sexual desire
> will experience short life. (However,) indulgence in sex will
> (also) result in failure to enjoy longevity. Only temperance
> in sexual activities can keep humans healthy in body and
> mind.[2]

---

[1] *Lao Lao Heng Yan (Perennial Sayings in Gerontology)*, quoted by Sun Guang-ren *et al.*, *Health Preservation and Rehabilitation*, Shanghai College of Traditional Chinese Medicine Press, Shanghai, 1990, p. 128

[2] Ge Hong, *Bao Pu Zi Nei Pian (Bao Pu-zi's Inner Writings)*, quoted by Sun Guang-ren *et al.*, *Ibid.*, p. 128

As discussed above, length of life is directly dependent upon the storage of *jing* essence in the kidneys. Besides prenatal and acquired *jing*, there is another kind of *jing* spoken of in Chinese medicine. This is the *sheng zhi zhi jing* or the reproductive essence. In men this refers to the semen and in women to the menstruate. This reproductive essence is lost to men in the act of ejaculation. Thus ejaculation in men directly affects the amount of their stored essence. When a man is young, they easily replace the essence lost in ejaculation. However, as one ages and their organs and bowels no longer function so efficiently, it becomes harder to manufacture abundant *qi* and therefore store *jing* essence.

Essence, Sex & Aging

Jing essence can be used for any of three purposes. It can be used for procreation, recreation, or transformation. Procreation means the making of babies. Recreation here means sexual pleasure. And transformation means spiritual transformation and physical rejuvenation. Above, we have said that a person is as old as their kidneys are, but this is just a way of saying that they are only as old as the amount of *jing* they have in store. *Jing* essence that is not used for procreation or recreation is used to repair and restore the physical body.

When I was young, we lived in a town where most of the people were Catholic, although my family was Protestant. Often, when I would be playing at my friends' houses, priests would visit to chat with their parents or to have supper. These men were an object of curiosity to me in part because I knew that they had taken a vow of perpetual celibacy. One of the things I noticed was how soft their skin was and how youthful they tended to look. Some might say that they looked young because they had relatively soft lives without the press and frustration of job and family. To some extent that probably did play a part in their smooth skin and youthfulness. However, when I later learned about the connection between the semen and the *jing* essence, their youthfulness and baby soft skin also became for me evidence of the validity of this connection. Later, when I became a Buddhist, I often had occasion to notice this same smoothness and youthfulness in Buddhist monks who had taken vows of celibacy.

Although some Chinese have taught that the road to immortality is by way of complete sexual abstinence, the safer and more natural approach is to pace one's sexual activity, timing it so that one has had an opportunity to replace any *jing* lost before losing it again. When attempting to erect (no pun intended) a schedule for ejaculation, there are several things to take into account. First is the constitution and health of the individual. A strong, robust man can ejaculate more frequently than a sick or weak one. Secondly, a younger man can ejaculate more frequently than an older man. And third, one can safely ejaculate more often in spring, less often in summer and fall, and perhaps not at all in winter if they are old or in poor health.

Pacing Ejaculation

Different Chinese sources give different schedules for ejaculation based on age. Typically, I suggest to my male patients that it is alright to have sex with ejaculation one to two times per day followed by a good night's sleep in their late teens and early twenties, once per day in their late twenties, once every other or third day in their thirties, once every week in their forties, once every twenty days in their fifties, and once a month or more in their sixties. However, men's sexual urge and sexual capacity differ and no one

43

schedule is right for all men. For this reason, Xu Ling-tai, a physician in the Qing dynasty (1644-1911 AD) advocated naturalness. Xu's idea of naturalness means to have sex only when one experiences a true and compelling build-up of the sexual urge. Most men as they enter their forties will experience diminished sexual desire. After sex, it takes several days or a week or so before that desire is felt again. After sex, older men may also experience fatigue, diminished strength, and lethargy. One should not have sex as long as these symptoms persist after sex. Nor should one have sex at the rate one has been having it if, after ejaculation, one experiences insomnia, agitations, dizziness, tinnitus, low back pain, or palpitations.

As for differences in the rate of sexual activity during the seasons, this is based on the Chinese idea of the seasons following a natural progression in the rise and fall of energy and, therefore, similarly of the energy within humans. In the spring, the energy is rested, restored, sprouting, and abundant. Therefore, the spring is the time of year when one can safely have the most sex. In the summer and fall, the energy is either at its peak or is already beginning to decline. Thus one's sexual activity should also begin to be curtailed. The winter, on the other hand, is a time of storage and quiescence. It is the season of the kidneys. That means it is the season that the kidneys need to recuperate and prepare for a new year. The Daoist master Liu Qing states:

> In spring one may shed *jing* once in these days, in the summer and autumn twice a month, but in winter, lock the *jing* and do not emit it. The *dao* of heaven is to store up

yang in the winter. If one can follow this, he will live a long time.[3]

It should also be mentioned that we are talking about sex with ejaculation. Sex without ejaculation can be had more frequently without detriment to the *jing* essence. However, one should not hold one's *jing* to the point of causing lower abdominal cramping. This can cause diseases of the urogenital tract which can also adversely affect the person's longterm health and longevity.

Women & Essence

All the above has been written from the perspective of the man. This is because men lose *jing* essence when they ejaculate in a way and amount which women do not. That does not mean sex does not consume *jing* in women. It does, but at a lesser amount. What does drastically consume *jing* in women is multiple pregnancies, pregnancy later in life, and prolonged breastfeeding or breastfeeding late in life. In addition, women's *jing* essence is also harmed by excessive menstrual bleeding, and menopause is the body's own wisdom curtailing the monthly lose of *jing* at the age when conservation of essence becomes a real issue.

Other Recommendations Concerning Sex

It also needs to be said that sex should not be had when intoxicated or when fatigued. When one is fatigued, ones' *qi* is already low. Loss of *jing* essence at that time only aggravates

---

3   Sun, James, "Pillars of Longevity", *Qigong, Health & Healing for the 21st Century*, Winter, 1993, p. 21

already deficient *qi* and impedes that *qi*'s recuperation. Alcohol is hot and acrid according to Chinese medicine. It injures both *yin* and *qi*. *Jing* essence is the root of both *yin* and *yang qi* in the body. If one loses their reproductive essence when their essence and qi are already decreased, this will likewise cause further detriment to the *qi* and *jing*. Nor should one indulge in sex when their stomach is too full or too empty. When the stomach is full, the *qi* accumulates in the stomach in order to transport and transform the food. Sex leads this *qi* away from the stomach and towards the kidneys and genitalia. Thus digestion is retarded and consequently so is *qi* production at a time when loss of essence makes *qi* production important. And when the stomach is empty and one is hungry, the *qi* is weak and needs to be replenished. As in the above instances, this is not the time to be losing one's *jing* essence.

Desire in Chinese medicine is a function of *yang qi*. Orgasm and ejaculation are a crescendo and climax of the growth of *yang* which then transforms into *yin*. Using Chinese herbs, it is possible to artificially stimulate this *yang qi* in order to stir up the sexual desire and achieve an erection when one is already satiated and fatigued from sex, drugs, alcohol, mental stress, or overwork. However, since such artificial stimulation only results in loss of *jing* when the body itself knows it does not have the juice to spare, such aphrodisiacs are ultimately bad for the health.

Once I had a patient who was in his late fifties. He had married in his twenties and this marriage had lasted for twenty years. In his late forties, he met a much younger woman who rekindled his sexual desire. He left his wife and had sex several times a day for a year or so. Little by little, however, this excessive sexual activity began to take its toll. At first he experienced premature ejaculation. This resulted in his

46

ejaculating even more frequently as he tried to satisfy his younger lover. Eventually he became impotent and his lover left him. I prescribed some Chinese herbs to replenish his *yang qi* and *jing* essence and told him that he shouldn't have any sex for three months. Unfortunately, I could not convince this man of the wisdom of these Chinese teachings on sexual moderation. As soon as he felt the stir of sexual arousal returning to his genitalia, he would watch pornographic movies and masturbate with a ring around the base of his penis to force an erection. He then could not understand why the Chinese treatment was not working. Eventually I suspended treatment since his abuse of these medicinals was only aggravating his condition.

The *Dao* of Sex

Readers familiar with the Chinese literature on sexual practices will undoubtedly have heard that men can increase their qi, health, and longevity and even achieve the *dao* by having a great deal of sex with numerous young nubile women as long as they do not ejaculate. This may, in fact, be true. However, such practices can lead to sexual vampirism even when their practice is technically correct and to disease and untimely death when practiced incorrectly or inappropriately. Zhu Dan-xi addresses this issue in his *Ge Zhi Yu Lun (Extra Treatises Based on Investigation & Inquiry)*:

> According to my understanding of the implication of the *Qian Jin ([Formulas Worth] a Thousand [Pieces of] Gold)* by Sun Si-miao, it is for those of robust age who are lustful and libidinous and whose water bodies are not so tranquil as before that the inner chamber method is designed as an aid to supplementation and boosting. This (art) can be applied (only) in those sturdy in physique with a tranquil

47

heart who can remain unstirred by an irresistible foe (*i.e.*, an attractive woman. This method) is not easy to perform for those without the heart of a sage or the bones of an immortal.[4]

Bedroom Taxation

In Chinese, strain due to excessive sexual activity is called *fang lao*, bedroom taxation. Sexual desire is the expression of abundant *yang qi* and *jing* essence. Sexual activity directly consumes and depletes this energy and essence. Moderate sex is extremely pleasurable and relaxing. Because it liberates pent up *qi*, moderate sex is even healthy and life-promoting. But excessive sex is one of the surest ways to cut one's life short. Several hundred years ago, the Daoist master Liu Qing wrote, "The affairs of the bedroom can give life to a man or it can kill him."[5] There is a Chinese story about an old man named Bao Hui who was 88 years old and who could still walk great distances without difficulty. When asked the secret of his longevity, he replied, "I have been taking a secret pill which can not be passed on to others." When asked what were the ingredients of this pill, Bao Hui answered, "I've been taking 'sleeping alone pills' for 50 years."

Zhu Dan-xi felt so strongly that inappropriate diet and sex are the two main impediments to achieving good health and long life that he begins his *Ge Zhi Yu Lun (Extra Treatises Based on*

---

4   Zhu Dan-xi, *Ge Zhi Yu Lun (Extra Treatises Based on Investigation & Inquiry),* translated by Yang Shou-zhong, Blue Poppy Press, Boulder, CO, to be released in 1994

5   Quoted by Sun, James, *op. cit.,* p. 21

Investigation & Inquiry) with a "Prologue to Admonitions on Food & Drink and Sexual Desire":

> It is stated in the *Zhuan (Commentaries [on the I Ching])* that human beings's great desires are for food and drink and sex. I often think to myself that desire for sex does (in fact) matter greatly and that desire for food and drink concerns the body particularly closely. In the world, there are not a few who, one after the other, become sunk deeply into such desires. If anyone really intends to devote themself to the *dao*, they must first take the study of this (problem) to heart.[6]

---

[6]   Zhu Dan-xi, *op. cit.*

5.

REST & RELAXATION

Although normal work and physical exercise are necessary to insure the circulation of *qi* and blood, to help the spleen and stomach generate *qi* and blood, and to build the body's ability to resist disease, every thought, word, and action does consume some amount of *qi* and *jing* essence. Every thought, word, and action is the manifestation of the movement of *qi* created by the transformation and consumption of *yin.* As long as we make more *qi* than we consume, we grow and flourish. However, by our mid-thirties, our digestion begins to weaken and we no longer make the abundant *qi* we once did from the food we eat and the air we breath. It becomes harder and harder to replace the *qi* we consume each day and, therefore, as we age, we must pay attention to sufficient rest and relaxation.

Physical Rest

Chapter 39 of the *Su Wen (Simple Questions)* states, "Overtaxation leads to qi exhaustion." Thus, when working, walking, or talking, it is important to stop and rest before one becomes too fatigued. This has to do with both prolonged exertion and overexertion, *i.e.,* doing something too long or doing something that is simply too much for one. Walking is relatively easy, but if one walks too long, they will become exhausted. However, trying to lift a very heavy object beyond the limits of one's strength can also be damaging to one's *qi*. As Sun Si-miao says, "It is desirable for one to frequently engage in minor jobs, without overfatiguing oneself by work so intense so as to exceed one's capabilities."[1] In particular, in modern, developed countries people work relatively long hours. Recently I read that in neolithic cultures, people only had to work approximately 20 hours per week to feed and shelter themselves. However, in so-called developed countries, people regularly work 40 and even more hours per week. Therefore, it is important for one to get adequate physical rest each day and also to take regular vacations throughout the year.

Economy of Speech

It is important for Westerners to understand that talking consumes great amounts of *qi*. In Chapter 1 above, we have discussed the creation of *qi* within the human organism. The body's *qi* is a combination of inhaled air and the finest essence of food and drink. This combination is made in the lungs and talking can immediately consume this *qi* at its source. Li Dong-yuan, in his *Pi Wei Lun (Treatise on the Spleen & Stomach)*, felt so strongly about the deleterious effects of over-speaking that he closed his last and greatest book with this admonition:

> Keep serene by all means, keep quiet by all means, and abide by natural law. A heavenly man (*i.e.*, an immortal)

---

[1] From Sun's *Qian Jin Yi Fang (Supplements to the Thousand [Pieces of] Gold)*, quoted by Sun Guang-ren *et al.*, *Health Preservation and Rehabilitation*, Shanghai College of Traditional Chinese Medicine Press, Shanghai, 1988, p. 122

can succeed in all of these. But what am I? It will be all right for me just to practice economy of speech.[2]

Sleep

Sleep is the greatest rest during the day. It is when all bodily functions slow down and when whatever surplus of *qi* and blood manufactured during the day has the opportunity to transform and be stored as *jing* essence. The amount of sleep necessary for any individual depends on their constitution, age, health, level of activity, and time of year. Most people do best sleeping during the night and working during the day since this corresponds to the relative proportions of *yin* and *yang* energy during those times. In Chinese medicine, sleep occurs when *yang qi* is embraced and enfolded by *yin qi*. As we age, we consume *yin qi* and this results in a relative excess of *yang* or active *qi*. Thus many people as they age have trouble with insomnia. They have become *yin* vacuous or deficient. Their *yin* is insufficient to hold down and enfold their *yang*. In this case, it is alright to nap during the day. It is also important to cultivate good sleeping habits.

There are three points to the Chinese teachings on developing good sleeping habits. These are keeping a calm mind, eating lightly before bed, and doing moderate exercise. Overexcitement or overthinking, which are expressions of the activity of *yang qi*, can affect the mind and keep one from sleeping. Therefore, one should try to calm the mind before attempting to fall asleep. The *Knack of Sleep* by Cai Ji-tong of

---

[2] Li Dong-yuan, *Li Dong-yuan's Treatise on the Spleen & Stomach, A Translation of the Pi Wei Lun*, trans. by Yang Shou-zhong, Blue Poppy Press, Boulder, CO, 1993, p. 261

the Song dynasty states that to sleep, first the mind must become calm and then the eyes.[3]

Secondly, one should not eat immediately before retiring for bed. The *yang qi* must retreat to the internal organs if one is to fall asleep. It does so by passing through several different layers of the body. One of these layers is the stomach. If the stomach is full of food, this *yang qi* gets stuck at this point and cannot retreat further to a state of unconsciousness.

And third, a little light exercise can help one go to sleep. Such exercise clears the mind of problems and circulates and pent-up *qi*. *The Secret of the Purple Rock* advises one to, "Walk 1,000 steps around the room before going to bed."[4] However, vigorous activities should be avoided, since they will cause difficulty in falling asleep.

Mental Tranquility

Not only does each physical movement and spoken word consume *qi*, but each sensation, each thought, and each feeling is the experience of the movement and transformation of *qi*. Because mental/emotional processes also consume *qi*, in fact great quantities of *qi*, it is not enough only to rest the body. If one is to live a long and healthy life, it is also important to adequately rest the mind. For Westerners, that may be even harder than practicing economy of speech.

---

[3]   Quoted by Yuan Li-ren & Liu Xiao-ming, "Traditional Chinese Methods of Health Preservation", *The Journal of Chinese Medicine*, UK, No. 41, Jan. 1993, p. 34

[4]   *Ibid.*, p. 34

There are innumerable methods of meditation and deep relaxation that seek to still the mind and calm the emotions. The key to all of these is mindfulness. Until one is aware that they are thinking unnecessary thoughts there is little way to diminish them. As one becomes aware that one is thinking, one can begin by trying to free their mind from unnecessary longing and wild fancy. Always wanting this or that, the mind never has a chance to settle and still itself. As soon as one becomes aware that they are thinking, the chain of thoughts breaks for a moment and there is space. If one becomes aware of their thoughts more and more often, this becomes a habit and there are more and more spaces where the mind can take rest.

In addition, because the body and mind are not two separate entities but are interdependent, one can calm the mind by relaxing the body. An up-tight mind usually goes hand in hand with muscular tension. The shoulders become raised, the eyebrows furrowed, the jaws clenched, and the breath held or restrained. As soon as one becomes aware of this holding and physical tension, one should exhale and let it go. It takes effort to hold this tension and all one has to do is become aware of it and release that tension. If one does that every day, day in and day out, one eventually becomes habituated to this process and can release tension and the thoughts behind that tension quite quickly.

Some Asian ascetics seek immortality by stopping the mental processes altogether. Whether this is even possible is subject to debate. However, it most definitely is true that a person can overthink and cause themselves fatigue and ill health. The signs of mental exhaustion due to overthinking include:

1. Dizziness, blurred vision, diminished hearing, and a burñing sensation in the ears
2. Weakness of the limbs, yawning, and sleepiness
3. Retardation of thought and reaction
4. Loss of appetite, nausea, and vomiting
5. Irritability, depression
6. Lack of comprehension when reading
7. Frequently misspelling or misspeaking oneself

Most of these symptoms have to do with either consumption of *qi* or consumption of *jing* essence. For instance, dizziness, blurred vision, diminished hearing, and burning ears all suggest kidney deficiency in Chinese medicine. While weakness of the limbs, fatigue, and loss of appetite are related to spleen *qi* vacuity or emptiness. Even if one is not trying to become a Daoist Immortal or even a centenarian, it is important to rest and relax if, through overwork and mental strain, one experiences any of these symptoms.

The word *si* in Chinese means to think, consider, or deliberate. However, it also means to long for. Thought is natural to humans but when it becomes excessive or obsessive, *i.e.*, worry, it becomes unhealthy. As Sun Guang-ren *et al.* say:

> According to TCM theory, man cannot go without thinking and remain idle. Deliberation within normal limits is beneficial instead of harmful; extreme deliberation for personal gains, which are always cherished in the mind but cannot be obtained with personal intelligence and wisdom, often result in disease.[5]

_____

[5]   Sun Guang-ren *et al.*, *op. cit.*, p. 124

Cao Ting-dong, author of the *Lao Lao Heng Yan (Perennial Sayings in Gerontology)*, opposed the Daoist and Buddhist ideas of complete mental inaction and aloofness from all mundane activities. He felt that, "The heart (*i.e.*, the mind) is not alright without something useful to apply itself to."[6] There is, however, a large and important difference in not doing anything and in practicing *qing jing wu wei* or peace, quiet, and not doing. This not doing is not doing anything contrary to natural law or the *dao*. Sun Si-miao clarified this when he said that in health preservation one should "not violate what their nature desires and move unhurriedly; not abandoning what is good to their ears and eyes, one accomplishes without difficulty."[7]

One very practical way of insuring one gets sufficient mental rest each day is to listen to a relaxation tape. Such tapes guide one's body and mind to successively deeper levels of relaxation. They require little self-discipline other than scheduling time each day to listen to the tape. If one does such a guided, progressive relaxation tape every day for 100 days, one will experience better energy, better mood, better digestion and elimination, and better sleep. A particularly good relaxation tape is *Chi Kung Meditations* by Ken Cohen, available from Blue Poppy Press.

_____

[6]   Quoted by Sun Guang-ren *et. al.*, *op. cit.*, p. 22

[7]   *Ibid.*, p. 12

6.

DAO YIN
SELF-MASSAGE

Qian Long's secrets 3-8 all have to do with a type of daily self-massage. This is called *dao yin* in Chinese. Literally, *dao yin* means to lead and guide. The implication is that through a combination of massage and visualization one can lead and guide their qi over the channels and connecting vessels of their body in a specific circuit. Qian Long's advice is to click the teeth together, swallow the saliva, massage the ears, rub the nose, roll the eyes, and knead the feet. This is but one self-massage or *dao yin* regimen recommended by Chinese longevity experts and below we will learn a similar but slightly expanded daily regime. However, first we should look at the reasons behind picking these particular areas of the body for self-massage.

In Chinese *yoga*, it is believed that the *qi* should run up the center of the back, over the top of the head, and down the center of the front of the body. On its ascent up the back, it follows what is called the governing vessel (*du mai*) which is also known as the sea of all *yang*. Down the front, it follows the path of the conception vessel (*ren mai*), the sea of all yin. This revolution up the back and down the front is called the microcosmic orbit. It is believed to mimic the ceaseless revolution and transformation of *yang* into *yin* into *yang* occurring in the world at large. By promoting this circuitous movement, one's *yin* and *yang* come into harmonious balance

59

like the smooth and perpetual workings of the heavens at large.

The mouth is the place where the governing and conception vessels meet. The governing vessel comes to an end in the teeth of the upper palate and the conception vessel takes up this flow of energy from the teeth and tongue of the lower palate. Both governing and conception vessels are believed to be connected and arise from out of the kidneys. In TCM, the teeth are said to be made from the surplus of the kidneys. Clicking the teeth stimulates the flow and interchange of *qi* from governing to conception vessel. Its vibrations also stimulate the brain which, in Chinese, is called the *sui hai*, sea of marrow. Marrow in Chinese is associated with the *jing* essence, and the brain is believed to be intimately connected with the *jing* essence of the kidneys.

The saliva is believed to be a very precious fluid according to the Chinese. In fact, Chinese medical theory posits the existence of two types of fluid in the mouth, one associated with the spleen and digestion and the other associated with the kidneys. Swallowing saliva accomplishes two things. According to Chen Ying-ning, it makes the turbid descend. This descent of the turbid in turn allows the arising of the clear *yang*, *i.e.*, the creation of *yang qi*, and results in spiritual brilliance (*shen ming*).[1] According to other Chinese authors, swallowing the saliva also returns the fluid associated with the kidneys back to the kidneys below to become *jing* essence.

---

[1]   Robert, Yves, "*Chen Yingning, un immortel dans le siecle*", *Medecine Chinoise & Medecines Orientales*, No. 4, Jan. 1993, p. 63

According to TCM theory, the ears, nose, and feet are all areas in which there is a *simulacrum* or *homunculus*. A *simulacrum* means a mirror image. A *homunculus* means a little person. What this means is that Chinese doctors believe there are maps or images of the entire body on each of these body parts. By stimulating these parts, one can stimulate the entire organism with all its organs and functions. It is as if each part of the body were a hologram of the entire body, that the entire body exists in each part. Certainly this is true from an embryological and genetic point of view. Chinese doctors have also identified other *homunculi* on the bones of the thumb and the thigh, on the face, and on the hands as well.

There are numerous different *dao yin* regimes in the Chinese longevity and *yoga* literature. Below is a regime I learned 15 years ago from a kung fu teacher. The number of repetitions specified for each movement are based on Chinese numerology. Basically, nine and its multiple as believed to be *yang* in nature and therefore healthful. Begin by sitting cross-legged on the floor. Loosen any belt or tight elastic around the abdomen. Rub the hands vigorously on the thighs creating a sense of heat and energy in the palms through friction. (Fig. 1) Then place the right palm on the lower abdomen covered by the left. Rub slowly back and forth from side to side across the lower abdomen. (Fig. 2) Do this 18 times. While doing this, imagine that there is a small incandescent sun at the level of the lower abdomen. This is called the lower *dan tian* or field of elixir where the *jing* essence is stored. Imagine that this rubbing causes this sun to glow more brightly and to emit more warmth. Think that this movement is like rekindling the coals sleeping under a bed of ashes. After 18 repetitions, pause for a moment with both hands over the lower *dan tian* and elbows pulled back to confirm the sensation of warmth in the lower abdomen.

Next slide the right hand out from under the left and around to rest palm down on the sacrum above the buttocks. The left hand should remain on the lower *dan tian*. Rub the sacral area to the left, down, to the right, and up in a continuous slow circle. (Fig. 3) Repeat this 18 times thinking that a line of light and warmth comes from the lower *dan tian*, passes in a loop around the base of the genitals and perineum, and runs up to the sacrum through the coccyx. Imagine the sacral area becoming warm and filled with light. At the end of 18 repetitions, pause with the right hand on the sacrum and cover it with the left hand. While pausing, mentally confirm this sensation/visualization.

Then slide the backs of both wrists up to the lumbar area on either side of the spine. Using the back of the wrists, rub in and down toward the spine and then out and up. (Fig. 4) Imagine light and warmth running up to the mid-lumbar area from the sacrum and that this light envelopes the kidneys, bathing them in energy and warmth. Do this 18 times. Then turn both palms down over the lumbar area covering the kidneys, pause, and confirm this sensation.

From the kidneys, place the palms of both hands loosely cupped over the ears with the fingers pointed back towards the base of the skull. Place each middle finger over the index finger and then flick the fingers producing a drumming on the base of the skull. (Fig. 5) This is called pounding the celestial drum. Repeat this 18 times. Take the hands off the ears and return them to the lap. Then click the teeth together vigorously 18 times. After that, raise the right hand to the top of the head and gently but firmly massage the gate to nirvana. (Fig. 6) This is the very top of the skull, midpoint between the ears and between the tip of the nose and base of the skull. Rub this area in a circular manner nine times.

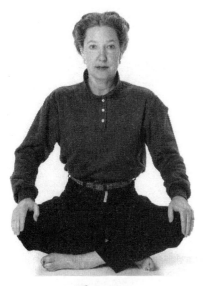

Figure 1

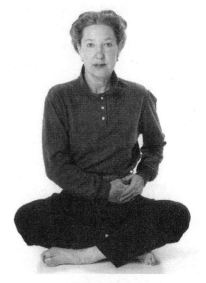

Figure 2

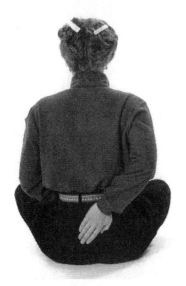

Figure 3

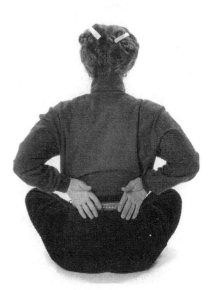

Figure 4

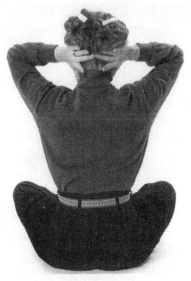

Figure 5

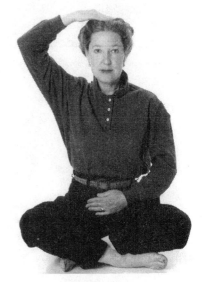

Figure 6

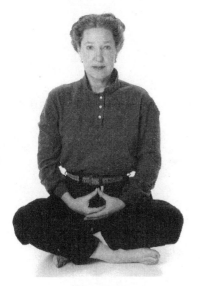

Figure 7

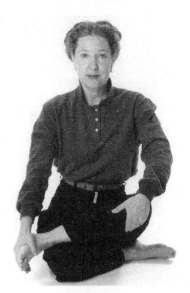

Figure 8

Let the right hand return to the lap. (Fig. 7) Next revolve
both the eyes and the tongue together nine times circling to
the right and nine times circling to the left. The tongue should
circle inside the teeth. The eyes may be either open or closed
depending upon whichever is easier. Saliva will be generated in
the mouth during this exercise, but this should not be
swallowed yet. Swish the saliva from front to back of the
mouth nine times thinking that by doing this the saliva is
energized. Then swallow the saliva in three measured gulps.
Imagine the saliva as a moonlike nectar which travels down
through the core of the body to the sun at the lower *dan tian*.
As it reaches the lower *dan tian*, it causes the sun to flare like
fat hitting a fire. Light and warmth then fill the entire body
out to every pore and part from the lower *dan tian*.

Next cross the right leg over the left knee. Place the right
palm on the right knee and the left palm on the sole of the
left foot. Rub slowly in a circular manner on both the knee
and sole simultaneously. (Fig. 8) Imagine that a line of light
runs from palm to palm traversing, warming, and energizing
the entire lower leg. Do this at least 18 times and up to 108
times. Then reverse and repeat the same this manueuvre with
the other leg. This concludes this particular *dao yin* regime. It
should take approximately 10 minutes to perform. One can
shorten the length of time it takes by reducing the number of
repetitions of each maneuver.

Each movement in the series has its own beneficial or
therapeutic effect. The set starts with rubbing the lower *dan
tian*. This corresponds to the sea of *qi* and chamber of essence.
Rubbing this area supplements this *qi* and essence which are
the roots of life.

65

Rubbing the sacrum assists the *yang*. A very strong flow of *yang qi* surfaces at the sacral hiatus to flow up the back and into the head. Rubbing the sacrum activates this *yang* energy. This *yang qi* is responsible for the functioning of the nervous system on one level and for spreading the defensive energy on another level. The sacrum is the root or foundation of the spinal column. It is also the pump of cerebrospinal fluid. As Western osteopaths and chiropractors have pointed out, the proper functioning and position of the spine is vitally important in maintaining the proper metabolism of the entire body.

Rubbing the lumbar region supplements of strengthens the kidneys. The kidneys are the most important organ in the body. They are the repository of the *jing* essence and the prenatal source *qi*. Rubbing this area primarily supplements kidney *yang* which is the source of fire or heat in the body. This area is also called the *ming men* or gate of life or destiny in Chinese. Kidney *yang* vacuity symptoms, such as impotence, polyuria, nocturia, tinnitus, and deafness due to old age, can be prevented in part through this maneuvre. Rubbing the kidneys can be performed at any time in the day as a separate therapy.

Pounding the celestial drum or the base of the skull strengthens the hearing, tonifies the brainstem and functions regulated by the brainstem, and relaxes the occipital region. Tension is this region can affect the flow of *yang qi* into the brain, the vision, and tension in the jaws. Tapping this area allows the *yang qi* to ascend unobstructed through the so-called window to the sky. It can help relieve tension headaches, chronic stiffness in the neck, and can also have a hypotensive effect.

Clicking the teeth also affects the gate at the back of the skull. The muscles from the jaws connect with the back of the skull. Therefore, clicking the teeth can reinforce the relaxing and opening promoted by pounding the celestial drum. In addition, clicking the teeth stimulates the central nervous system by vibrating the brain and as well as strengthens the teeth and gums. It helps prevent bleeding gums and loose teeth.

Acupuncturists refer to the crown of the head as the meeting of hundreds (*bai hui*). It is the reunion point for all the *yang* channels in the body. It is the microcosmic North Star of the body. From a medical point of view, stimulation of this meeting of hundreds raises clear *yang*, calms the spirit, and clears the mind. It also helps to regulate the central nervous system in general. In Buddhism, this point is called the gate to nirvana. Its opening is essential in yogic practices of ejecting the consciousness at the moment of death.

Rotating the eyes strengthens the vision. Besides, the eyes are an outgrowth of the brain. Rotating the eyes, therefore, can stimulate the entire central nervous system. Energetically, it effects the flow of energy to and through the pituitary.

The tongue is the "sprout of the heart" according to Chinese medicine and is also connected to the spleen and stomach. Rotating the tongue stimulates the digestion, the root of postnatal *qi* and blood production. As mentioned above, many Chinese have viewed saliva as a type of internal elixir. Some people believe it has an anticarcinogenic effect. Yogically, saliva is a "lunar" nectar. Bringing that nectar down to the sun of the lower *dan tian* is believed to create an inner elixir which can tonify and transform the entire body.

67

Rubbing the feet stimulates the kidney *yin* energy, our connection with the earth, *i.e.,* material existence. Just as rubbing the crown of the head stimulates our connection with heaven, this *yang* energy must be led downward again to maintain the balance between *yin* and *yang* or form and function. As mentioned above, rubbing the feet can strengthen the energy of the entire body, since the feet contain a reflex map of the entire body. Further, by rubbing the feet with the hands, one is leading the energy out into all four limbs. Bringing the *qi* up the back and down the front of the torso is called the microcosmic orbit. Circulating that energy out into the feet and hands as well completes what is called the macrocosmic orbit, thus ensuring the flow of *qi* and blood to the entire body.

Different practitioners may give the different moves different names and may specify different numbers of strokes on each point based on numerological biases inherent in different philosophical schools. The important thing is regularity and perserverence in its practice. Other specific self-massage maneuvers can be added if they do not violate the flow of the sequence depending upon their need or other strokes may be appended afterward to remedy specific situations. Typically, such *dao yin* regimes are done upon arising in the morning. They are easy to do and do not require strength or youthful stamina. However, they are based on profound theories and many generations of Asian practitioners' experiences.

7.

EXERCISE & STRETCHING

The *Nei Jing* states, "Prolonged sitting damages the flesh" and "Prolonged lying damages the qi." For not less than 2,000 years Chinese doctors have believed that lack of adequate physical exercise leads to disease. As a modern Chinese acupuncture text says, "Lack of physical exercise can impair the circulation of *qi* and blood, weaken the function of the spleen and stomach, and sap body resistance."[1] When we exercise, the rhythmic contraction and release of our muscles, the increased pumping of our heart, and the expansion and contraction of our lungs all promote the flow and circulation of *qi*, blood, and body fluids. This increased circulation of *qi* results in the upbearing of the clear and downbearing of the turbid. In Chinese medical terms, this implies that digestion is improved. When digestion is improved, *qi* and blood production also improves. And abundant *qi* and blood result in increased immunity to disease.

In developed countries, due to sedentary lifestyle and labor-saving devices, many people do not get enough physical exercise. Because many people in such countries also suffer from increased job and lifestyle stress, this lack of adequate exercise is doubly harmful. The manifestations of inadequate

---

[1] *Chinese Acupuncture and Moxibustion*, ed. by Cheng Xin-nong, Foreign Languages Press, Beijing, 1987, p. 249-250

exercise are softening of the bones and tendons, lack of energy, poor appetite, lassitude, obesity, and shortness of breath on exertion. Psychologically, lack of exercise also exacerbates anxiety, irritability, and depression. Although much of the Chinese longevity literature seems to emphasize not overworking and overtaxing oneself, Chinese longevity experts have also recommended avoiding excessive comfort. Lu Jiu-zhi of the Qing dynasty, in his *Yi Bing Lun (Treatise on Leisure Diseases)* pointed out that, "Ordinary people are often told of diseases from overtaxation but have no knowledge of diseases due to excessive leisure; the latter, however, are more harmful."[2] Liu goes on to say,

> If ordinary people remain idle and unoccupied, this leads to disease. If minor labor returns one's strength, if their disease improves when occupied by affairs and when busy they can forget their disease, if they feel fatigued after meals or fatigued after sleep, this is leisure disease.[3]

Essentially, humans need regular physical exercise. However, that exercise should be moderate, not too much and not too little. Too much and *qi* and blood are consumed in excess. Too little and *qi* and blood are not produced and do not circulate. The famous Han dynasty doctor, Hua Tuo, said,

> The human body desires work and movement, but one should not exert themself to the extreme. Movement of the body leads to grain *qi* being completely dispersed. The

---

[2]   Quoted by Sun Guang-ren *et al.*, *Health Preservation and Rehabilitation*, shanghai College of Traditional Chinese Medicine Press, Shanghai, 1988, p. 142

[3]   *Ibid.*, p. 142

blood vessels flow freely. And disease cannot arise. This is like a (leather) door hinge which never becomes rotten.[4]

In the Tang Dynasty, Sun Si-miao reiterated this same teaching, "The body desires labor, but one should never labor to extreme."[5] Because one's strength, energy, and condition vary from day to day, season to season, and from age to age, this means that one should also regulate their exercise to meet their own particular needs. When one is young and in the prime of their life, doing strenuous physical exercises is appropriate. However, as one ages, one's exercise can and should become milder and less strenuous. Exercise which results in a person feeling exhausted afterwards is too much.

For the purposes of this discussion, there are five kinds of exercise:

1. Physical exercise which is a part of living one's life
2. Aerobic exercise
3. Resistance training
4. Stretching
5. *Qi gong*

Doing Chores by Hand

Physical exercise which is a part of living one's life refers to the walking, moving, and lifting inherent in just moving through one's daily schedule. In undeveloped countries, daily life for most people is made up of a series of physical tasks. One typically must walk everywhere. Stairs need to be climbed. Water needs to be carried or pumped. Wood or brush

---

4   *Ibid.*, p. 8

5   *Ibid.*, p. 142

71

needs to be carried for fuel. Dishes and clothes need to be washed by hand. The garden needs to turned, planted, weeded, and harvested. One's house needs to be cleaned.

In rich, Western countries, many of these simple physical tasks have been replaced by machines and appliances. In such countries, one of the easiest ways of getting adequate exercise is to forego the use of one's car, elevator, and other mechanical conveniences and chose instead to do these things manually or by one's own body. Instead of driving everywhere, sometimes one should walk or ride their bicycle. Instead of taking the elevator, one should walk up the stairs. This kind of exercise is relatively easy to do since it is purposeful and uncontrived.

Aerobic Exercise

Some people just cannot find the time to walk to work or get their exercise entirely by doing manual chores during their daily schedule. In that case, it is necessary to set time aside to deliberately exercise. There are three types of exercise a person should do in order to stay healthy. The first of these is aerobic exercise. This means doing something fast enough and repetitive enough to get one's heart beating 80% faster than normal. This means that if one's normal resting pulse is 72 beats per minute, one's aerobic rate should be at least 128 beats per minute. Once one's rate is up to that point, one then needs to keep it there for a continuous 20 minutes.

This can be accomplished by fast walking, jogging, riding a bicycle, swimming, playing basketball, or any of a number of other methods of exertion. The exact method is not that important as long as one's heart beat is raised and one keeps that rate up for 20 minutes to a half hour. The important thing other than that is that whatever method of exercise one chooses should not cause any damage to any part of the body.

72

Since many types of aerobic exercise consist of doing the same movements over and over again repetitively, if those movements are even just a little bit damaging to the joints and tendons, a host of small injuries may accumulate to result in a large problem. Therefore, one should chose an aerobic activity which will not result in cumulative stress injuries, or one should vary the type of aerobic activity so as not to always stress the same body parts.

Aerobic exercise results in circulating the *qi*, blood, and body fluids. It strengthens the heart and lungs and reduces the negative effects of stress and emotional strain. Young and middle-aged people should do some kind of aerobic activity at least three times per week.

Resistance Training

Resistance training refers to lifting or pushing against something heavy or difficult to move. Resistance training builds physical strength. It also converts fat into muscle. Muscle burns more calories than does adipose or fatty tissue. When one reaches 40 years of age, one's metabolism naturally slows down with the decline of organ functions. Practically speaking, this results in gaining approximately 10 pounds every decade after that age unless one takes preventive steps. After 40, one will gain weight even if one eats the same amounts and kinds of foods and gets the same amount of exercise they did before that age. In other words, in order to counteract this process, one has to do more than they did before.

Lifting weights, doing push-ups, sit-ups, and pull-ups, or using any of the numerous types of resistance training machines on the market can help convert fatty tissue into muscle. Not only will this result in a slimmer, trimmer body, but one will also feel mentally and emotionally good about their renewed physical strength. They will feel strong and robust and young. The old saying goes, "Nothing succeeds like success." If, through resistance training, one becomes pleased by their youthful body in comparison to others their same age who have not taken such good care, this healthy pride and positive self-image can help develop more *joie de vivre* and with that a longer, healthier life.

When doing resistance training, one should exercise all major muscle groups. One should not try to build huge muscles but rather concentrate on toning and firming what they have. This usually means lighter weights or less resistance and more repetitions. Resistance training can be done three or more times per week but should be done at least twice a week. Besides the benefits mentioned above, resistance training also results in stronger bones and tendons.

Stretching

In the *Huai Nan Zi*, a compilation of philosophical treatises commissioned by Prince Huai Nan in the 2nd century BC, it says: "A pure spirit, emotions in equilibrium, and relaxation of all the joints are basic for the sustenance of one's essential nature."[6] In Chinese medicine, the joints are seen as areas where there is a special concentration of *qi* and blood. From the traditional Chinese point of view, this is why movement occurs at the joints. These are the places where the sinews attach to the bones and where the channels and connecting vessels flow close to the skin, sandwiched closely between both. Although the joints are places where the *qi* and blood should flow most freely, in fact, they are places where the *qi* and blood can become easily stuck or stagnant.

---

[6] Quoted by Manfred Porkert, *Theoretical Foundations of Chinese Medicine*, MIT Press, Cambridge, MA, 1982, p. 20

Stretching exercises help to loosen the joints and promote the free flow of *qi* and blood over the channels and connecting vessels. They strengthen the tendons and ligaments and also indirectly strengthen the bones. Further, stretching exercises help promote mental and physical relaxation.

Stretching exercises are easiest to do in the late afternoon or early evening and are hardest to do in the early morning when one first wakes up. However, doing stretching exercises in the morning helps to free the flow of *qi* and blood which has become sluggish overnight. When doing stretching exercises, it is important to relax into each stretch. One should work with their breath, relaxing further with each exhalation. One should not try to stretch by bouncing into a stretch, nor should they force themselves to stretch too far too fast. Rather, one should stretch little by little, day by day, making haste slowly.

Many systems of Chinese martial arts teach stretching exercises. However, one does not have to take a class at their local *kung fu* studio to learn how to stretch. The most important stretches are to flex and extend the spine, to adduct the spine, and to rotate the spine. Also, one should stretch out the backs of the legs which tend to be tight. One can also stretch their legs apart as if attempting a split. For more information on stretching, the reader should see Bob Anderson's classic, *Stretching*.[7] Stretching should be done on a daily basis in order to keep the body supple, the *qi* and blood flowing freely, and the mind relaxed.

Qi Gong

The following chapter is devoted to the fifth type of exercise described in this book. *Qi gong* can mean many different

---

[7]   Anderson, Bob, *Stretching*, Shelton Publications, Bolinas, CA, 1980

things to different people. Many Chinese refer to almost all stretching exercises and calisthenics as *qi gong*. However, since the word itself means to train or discipline the *qi*, I differentiate it from stretching, calisthenics, and self-massage. As one ages, one does not need and indeed should not do the heavy exercise one was capable of as a young or middle-aged adult. *Qi gong* exercises are a way of getting moderate exercise without excessive strain. As middle age gives way to old age, it is probably better for most people to combine *qi gong* with stretching exercises and then to be sure they stay physically active in their daily routine.

Although one must moderate their exercise with advancing age, it is nonetheless important not to stop exercising. One of the characteristics of *qi* within the human body is movement. The body stops moving when the *qi* departs. But if one stops moving, one's *qi* will depart all the quicker.

8.

QI GONG

Qi gong means to train or discipline one's *qi*. According to Ken Cohen, a well known *qi gong* teacher in the West, this term did not come into use in China until 1934.[1] However, what we today call *qi gong* has been practiced in China since not less than 400 BC. In the 1970's, a series of tombs were excavated in China at a site called Ma Wang Dui near Changsha. These contained a cache of books written on bamboo slats and silk rolls. A number of these books were on medical subjects. Amongst these books were pictures of various exercises believed to confer health benefits and contribute to longevity. At approximately the same time, the great Daoist philosopher, Zhuang Zi, wrote about such exercises and their healing properties.

During the Han dynasty (25-220 AD), a scholar named Wei Bo-yan wrote a book on what has now come to be known as *qi gong*. Titled *Chan Tong Qi (Three in One)*, it discusses the relationship between Daoism, the *Yi Jing (Classic of Changes)*, and *qi gong*. Wei was the first Chinese to write about *qi gong* from the perspective of the *jing* essence, *qi*, and *shen* spirit.

---

[1]   Cohen, Ken, "*Qigong*, Cultivating the Vital Breath", *Qi, The Journal of Traditional Eastern Health & Fitness*, Vol. 1, No. 2, Summer, 1991, p. 23. According to Cohen, the first use of this term in the Chinese literature appears in Dong Hao's *Special Treatments for Lung Diseases: Qigong Treatments*.

Also during the Han dynasty, Hua Tuo, perhaps the most famous doctor in Chinese created his Five Animal Frolics. This was a series of *qi gong* exercises based on mimicking the movements and breath patterns of five different animals known either for their strength or longevity. These exercises are still taught and practiced to this day. Hua Tuo lived to be 97 at which time he was executed. He was still married when he died. His two students, Fan Ao and Wu Chin lived to be 100 plus and 90 years old respectively.

During the next 1,700 years, according to the *Dao Shu (Daoist History)*, 3,600 different kinds of *qi gong* developed. According to Gan Zhen-yun, "The main features of Qigong development in this stage were: the widespread application of Qigong for health protection and medical care, and its integration with Chinese medicine which promoted the development of traditional medical science."[2] In more modern times, Zhang Zi-yang wrote several books on *qi gong* and health preservation, including *Understand the Truth, 400 Characters on Qi Gong*, and *Secrets for Keeping One's Youth*. In these books, Zhang further developed, enriched, and perfected the theories on the relationship of *qi gong* to the *jing, qi*, and *shen* first advanced by Wei Bo-yan 900 years before.

As mentioned above, there are many different styles of *qi gong* and literally thousands of different *qi gong* exercises. However, most *qi gong* exercises are based on the coordination of three elements: 1) a specific pattern of breathing, 2) a specific posture or movements coordinated with that breath pattern, and 3) a visualization accompanying both breath pattern and movements or posture. As we have seen above, one's *qi* is manufactured in part from the purest essence of the air we

---

[2]   Gan Zhen-yun, "The History of Chinese Qigong", *Qi, The Journal of Traditional Eastern Health & Fitness*, Vol. 3, No. 3, Autumn, 1993, p. 21

breath. Through *qi gong* exercises we can manufacture *qi* more efficiently, store *qi* more effectively, and circulate our *qi* more smoothly. In addition, we can circulate our *qi* to particular places or organs in our body to bath those areas in healing, revitalizing energy.

In China there are Confucian styles of *qi gong*, Daoist styles of *qi gong*, and Buddhist styles of *qi gong*, each with their own unique theories and techniques. In addition, many *qi gong* exercises are associated with Chinese martial arts, such as *Tai Ji Quan, Ba Gua Zhang,* and *Xing Yi Quan.* Further, there are also types of medical *qi gong* specifically meant for the healing of disease or increasing one's health. *Qi gong* has become extremely popular, even faddish, in China in the last dozen years or so, and there are many books available on this subject in both Chinese and English. There are even a number of video tapes available to help one learn *qi gong.*

Generally, it is best to study *qi gong* as part of a class under the guidance of a qualified instructor. *Qi gong* instruction is now available in all large cities and many medium sized cities in the United States. However, to get a taste of *qi gong* and to literally feel one's *qi*, I give instructions on how to do a simple *qi gong* exercise below. But, before immediately jumping to that exercise, it is important to mention a couple of more introductory things about this ancient Oriental exercise art.

First, *qi gong* emphasizes deep, abdominal breathing. Such deep diaphragmatic breathing rids the lungs of stale air and bathes the organism in fresh air. In addition, this deep breathing has a massaging effect on the internal organs and promotes the flow of blood, lymph, and cerebrospinal fluids. Secondly, the breath associated with most *qi gong* exercises has four characteristics. It is long, thin, even, and slow. It is not hurried, choppy, coarse, or rough. This relaxed, rhythmic, deep breathing thus helps calm the mind and relieves stress.

79

And secondly, *qi gong* involves concentrating the mind and ridding it of distracting thoughts. In Chinese this is called *shou yi*. *Shou* means to concentrate, to attend to, or to look after. *Yi* means one. Thus *shou yi* means to concentrate on only one thing. During *qi gong*, such one-pointed concentration can be on a point within or part of the body, on the breath, or on a visualization or sensation. As Wang Zhi-xing, a *qi gong* teacher active in England and Europe says:

> *Shou yi* teaches us to rest our mind internally on the oneness instead of restlessly jumping from one idea to the next. *Shou yi* helps us settle our mind and spirit internally and to focus our senses deeply within instead of looking outward all the time. *Shou yi* guides us to integrate ourselves with our circumstances and helps us to relax in different situations. Through *shou yi*, one's mind becomes peaceful and empty; the body, mind, and spirit are harmonized and the *shen* is therefore pacified and nourished.[3]

Rising Eagle

The following is a very simple *dong gong* or moving *qi gong* exercise. It helps to circulate the *qi*, store the *qi* and *jing* essence in the lower *dan tian*, and rids the lungs of stale air. It is a good exercise to do on waking in the morning as per Qian Long's suggestion.

Begin by standing erect with feet planted shoulder width apart. The head and torso should be erect. The butt and hips should be allowed to release and slide forward, thus straightening out the curve of the low back. In addition, the knees should be

---

[3] Wang Zhi-xing, "The Cultivation of *Shen* with *Qigong*", *The European Journal of Oriental Medicine*, Vol. 1, No. 1, Spring, 1993, p. 35

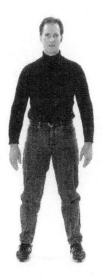

Figure 1

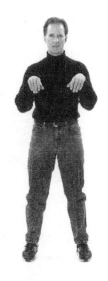

Figure 2

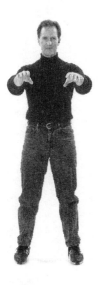

Figure 3

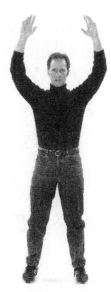

Figure 4

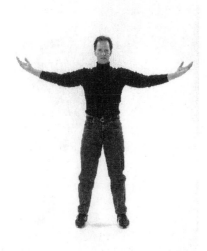

Figure 5

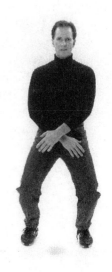

Figure 6

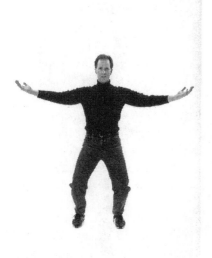

Figure 7

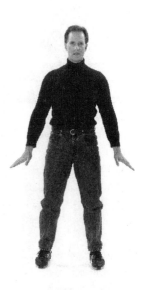

Figure 8

slightly bent and the weight should be evenly distributed over the entire foot, leaning neither on the heels or the balls and toes. Relax the shoulders and let the arms hang to one's side with the fingers gently extended. (Fig. 1) The breath should be through the nose with the mouth gently shut. Breathe in by expanding the lower abdomen and breathe out by contracting the lower abdomen. As one breathes, let the feeling of the mind, the feeling of consciousness sink to the lower *dan tian*. This is a spot 3-4 inches below the navel and a third of the way into the body. One should try to keep their mind fixed in this place or space and do the following exercise from the lower *dan tian*.

As one breathes in, let the wrists float up to the level of the chest. (Fig. 2) Feel as if there were a string attached to the wrists picking up the arm from that point. As the wrists reach the level of the chest, begin exhaling and let the hands move forward until the arms are almost straight out in front of one. (Fig. 3) Then breathe in and let the hands and arms float up over one's head. (Fig. 4) Breathe out and sink slowly into the knees as the arms move out to the sides and down. (Fig. 5) Keeping the knees bent, the hands move down and across the legs, left hand passing over right. (Fig. 6) As the hands swing apart again, begin to breathe in but do not straighten the legs. One should remain with their knees bent and buttocks tucked underneath their hips. (Fig. 7) As the hands reach the level of the shoulders, one turns their palms over so that they are facing downward. Then exhaling, the hands push down as one rises from their bent position. (Fig. 8) Again the wrists are drawn up towards the level of the chest as one breathes in and the entire exercise is repeated.

When doing this exercise there are a number of things to keep in mind. First, the mind leads the breath, the breath leads the *qi*, and it is the *qi* that leads the motion. The *qi* goes where the mind and breath lead it. That's why what we call moving *qi gong* today was simply part of what was called *dao yin*, or leading and guiding. As one moves, feel as though the air is as thick as water. Try to move very slowly with one motion blending into the next. Try to accomplish each movement with the minimal amount of physical strain or effort. Let the entire body remain relaxed yet erect as if suspended from a string tied to the crown of the head. Repeat this exercise 9 times.

As one completes the ninth repetition, let the arms come back to the resting position and just stand for a moment. One should feel relaxed but energized. The body should feel transparent but at the same time very full. Perhaps one feels a lot of tingling in their fingers and their hands feel slightly swollen and enlarged. These are all immediate, felt experiences of one's *qi*. Visualize this *qi* filling one's body like mist in a bottle. But visualize it as a mist made out of light. Then imagine this mist of light seeps into the heads of the bones, filling the bones with bright, incandescent lasers or filaments of light. Think that one has locked their *qi* into their bones, fusing it with their marrow and that their bones thus become diamond hard and filled with essence. Then swallow any saliva filling the mouth in three measured swallows and visualize this saliva travelling down to the lower *dan tian*. As the saliva reaches the lower *dan tian*, imagine that warmth and light is generated from that spot radiating out and enlivening the entire rest of the body.

This exercise helps to expel stale air from the lungs and gently circulates the qi through the entire body. It is best to do this exercise in a room with an open window. If one does this exercise outside, one can also practice facing the rising sun and, in that case, also visualize one absorbing the *yang qi* and warmth of the sun as they inhale. One can also do this exercise after doing *dao yin* self-massage instead.

Hu Bin, in *A Brief Introduction to the Science of Breathing*, describes the following eight common, normal reactions to *qi gong* practice. These are:

1. Profuse secretion of saliva
2. Improved sense of mental clarity
3. Improved and sound sleep
4. Warm sensations in various body parts
5. Better digestion and improved appetite
6. Light itching and involuntary muscular contractions
7. Active body metabolism as evidenced by increased normal bodily secretions and faster growth of hair, nails and beard
8. Mental and physical relaxation and a sense of harmony and ease[4]

All these signs and symptoms show that healthy organ function is increased, there is abundant *qi* and blood, and that *yin* and *yang* are in harmonious balance.

Qi gong can be very powerful and it is best to learn *qi gong* from a qualified instructor. It is important not to strain when doing *qi gong*, not to do too much *qi gong*, and not to do *qi gong* immediately after a meal. If one experiences headaches, pain in the chest or ribs, pain or stuffiness below the ribs, or abdominal distention, one is either doing too much *qi gong* or is not relaxing enough. These are symptoms of *qi* stagnation. In this case, one should stop doing *qi gong* and see either a *qi gong* instructor or Chinese doctor or both.

---

[4] Hu Bin, *A Brief Introduction to the Science of Breathing*, Hai Feng Publications, Hong Kong, 1983, p. 77

9.

CHINESE HERBAL MEDICINE

So-called herbal medicine is the main modality in Traditional Chinese Medicine. I say so-called because Chinese herbal medicine uses medicinals from all three kingdoms—plant, animal, and mineral. Thus traditional Chinese internal medicine uses more than just herbs. One of Qian Long's secrets for longevity is the regular use of supplementing medicinals. In Chinese medicine, practitioners have identified a number of ingredients which supplement or tonify the *qi* and blood and *yin* and *yang*. The wise use of these supplementing ingredients can slow down the aging process and help maintain a healthy, vigorous old age.

As we age, *qi* and blood production decline due to the weakening of organ function in general and of our digestion in particular. Thus the organism must dip into its reserves of *jing* essence more and more. At first, people become relatively *yin* deficient or vacuous. Our skin becomes dry and wrinkles appear. Our hair turns white and even falls out due to *yin* and blood vacuity failing to nourish the hair. Further, loss of hearing and visual acuity and a tendency to insomnia, all characteristic of aging, are all due to decline and insufficiency of *yin* blood. Women's menstruation ceases and they may experience vaginal dryness and atrophy. Even weakening of the bones and loss of height have to do with this progressive consumption of *yin jing* and the drying out it entails.

Eventually, however, we become so *yin* deficient that *yang* also starts to decline. This is because *yang* is rooted in, nourished by, and created out of *yin* substance. When *yang* likewise becomes weak and deficient, we catch cold easily, sleep a lot during the day, our hands and feet are hard to keep warm, we lose our strength and our energy, and we urinate too frequently. We especially lose our sexual desire or at least see it significantly diminish, and men lose the ability to gain and maintain an erection.

Further, as *qi* and blood decline, the blood and body fluids fail to circulate freely as they should. It is the *qi* which moves the blood and body fluids. If the *qi* is weak, it cannot move and transport the blood and body fluids which then accumulate and form stagnation and stasis. In addition, if the blood is deficient, it may be insufficient to fill and keep open the channels and vessels and for this reason also blood stasis may occur. For instance, so-called liver or age spots are believed to be the result and manifestation of static blood in the superficial blood vessels, and diseases such as prostatic hypertrophy in the elderly are commonly diagnosed in TCM as blood stasis.

Superior, Medium, & Inferior Grade Herbs

The traditional Chinese pharmacopeia or list of medicinal substances is comprised of 5,762 ingredients.[1] Since the 600's, these have been divided into three grades. The superior grade of medicinals is believed to generally nourish life, *yang sheng*. This category is composed of *qi*, blood, *yin*, and *yang* supplements which literally help the body make more of each

_____

[1]   *Zhong Yao Da Ci Dian (The Encyclopedia of Chinese Medicinals)*, Shanghai Science and Technology Press, Shanghai, 1991

of these. These medicinals do not so much eliminate disease as boost the body's own vitality. They are non-toxic and can be used preventively and long term even by those who show no sign of disease. The most famous example of a superior grade medicinal for the nourishment of life is ginseng, which is believed to supplement the *qi*, nourish the blood, and fortify the essence.

The second category of medicinals, the medium grade, is composed of ingredients that nourish the form or body, *yang xing*. These medicinals are mostly non-toxic or have little toxicity. These medicinals are used to treat light or chronic diseases. These medicinals can be used frequently but not as freely as the superior grade. Their use should be based on a professional TCM diagnosis. Ingredients in this category include bupleurum and pinellia.

The third category of medicinals, the lower grade, is composed of ingredients which have some definite element of toxicity. These medicinals are only to be used if one is diseased. Specifically, they are said to expel disease, or *zhu bing*. They are for the remedial treatment of more acute, serious, and even potentially life-threatening diseases. When such toxic medicinals are used, they should be suspended as soon as they have achieved their effect. Prolonged use of this grade of medicinals results in harm to the body and its *qi* and blood. Ingredients in this category include realgar, *i.e.*, arsenic trisulfide, euphorbia, and poke root.

Animal "Herbs"

Many of the tonic or supplementing category of traditional Chinese medicinals are made from animals, and many of these sound quite exotic to modern Western ears. These include

89

seahorses and sea dragons or pipefish, turtle and tortoise shell, deer and seal testicles, deer antler, tiger bone, human placenta, gecko lizards, and donkey skin gelatin. It is said that animal medicinals are more compassionate to the human body than vegetable medicinals. This means that they are both stronger for supplementing the *qi*, blood, *yin*, and *yang* and that they are closer in form to the human body itself. Thus many of the tonic formulas designed to restore or maintain youthfulness are made from such exotic animal ingredients.

In recent years, another animal medicinal which has gained great popularity as a tonic in both the East and West is royal bee jelly. This is the jelly feed by worker bees to the queen bee and accounts for the queen bee's longevity and ability to lay thousands and thousands of eggs. Like other of the animal tonics, royal jelly is believed to be a powerful *yin* and blood supplement. Many other tonic medicinals are prepared with royal jelly for easy, tasty, daily consumption, such as ginseng and royal jelly and deer antler and royal jelly.

Plant Medicinals

However, not all Chinese longevity medicinals are made from animal parts and pieces. Many Chinese herbs are known for their ability to nourish life. The most famous of these in the West is probably ginseng. This root is believed by Chinese doctors to greatly supplement the original energy of the individual. In Chinese, it is called *Ren Shen* or Human Root. Although it supplements the *qi* of the spleen, lungs, and kidneys in particular, it also supplements all the organs in the body and nourishes the blood as well. Old people in China typically take a course of ginseng in the winter months. It can be taken as a tea, with wine, or even simply eaten.

Another famous Chinese longevity herb is *He Shou Wu* or Mr. He's Black Hair. This is the root of Polygonum Multiflorum. It is sometimes also referred to as *Fo Ti*. It got its name because a Mr. He supposedly started eating this herb late in life after his hair had already begun to turn white. After some time, his neighbors saw that his hair had turned black and lustrous again and that he remained youthful and robust. He is even believed to have fathered children well into his 80's and all due to the regenerative and restorative powers of this root. Nowadays, this root is categorized as blood and liver and kidney supplement in TCM.

Chinese Patent Medicines

Various pharmaceutical companies in China manufacture a large number of prepared or so-called patent medicines. These are meant for over the counter consumption and many of them are specifically composed of supplementing medicinals. These patent medicines come mostly as pills but also as wines. Because old age is a chronic condition, supplementing medicinals need to be taken day in and day out, and pills and wines are much easier to take than boiling up the traditional Chinese decoction from bulk herbs. *The Dao of Increasing Longevity and conserving Life: A Handbook of Traditional Chinese Geriatrics and Chinese Herbal Patent Medicines*[2] written by Anna Lin and myself is a book entirely on the subject of using Chinese patent medicines for the treatment of the most common diseases associated with aging and for nourishing life in general.

---

[2] Lin, Anna & Flaws, Bob, *The Dao of Increasing Longevity and Conserving One's Life: A Handbook of Traditional Chinese Geriatrics and Chinese Herbal Patent Medicines*, Blue Poppy Press, Boulder, CO, 1991

Seeking a Professional Prescription

All the other regimes discussed in this book can be done without recourse to health care professionals. They are free therapies in that they do not cost anything but one's time and commitment. In the last 10 years, Chinese herbs and Chinese patent medicines have become widely available in Western health food stores. However, although Chinese tonic medicinals tend to be non-toxic from the traditional Chinese point of view, they are not entirely safe when self-prescribed by the layperson.

As mentioned above, some medicinals supplement the *qi* and others nourish the blood. Yet others strengthen *yang* and still others enrich *yin*. Chinese medicine is based on the concept of harmony. Health is seen as just the right amounts and proportions of *qi* and blood, *yin* and *yang*. If a person takes the wrong supplement medicinals, these can cause an imbalance and, because of that imbalance, lead to the creation or aggravation of disease. In some cases, already established diseases must be treated first before one should use supplementing and tonifying medicinals. Even the Chinese herbal medicinals meant for nourishing life are not panaceas or cure alls.

Therefore, it is important especially for Westerners who have not grown up with the concepts and medicinals of TCM to seek a professional prescription for their Chinese herbs. If a person is primarily *qi* deficient, their TCM practitioner will prescribe the appropriate *qi* supplements. But if they are blood deficient, their TCM practitioner will prescribe the appropriate blood-nourishing herbs. In particular, if one is *yin* vacuous and they take a *yang* supplement, this will make their *yin* vacuity even worse. Also, if they have blood stasis, supplementing the *qi* and blood without first removing this stasis may make that stasis worse. Thus it is my strong advice to only take Chinese herbal medicinals from professional TCM practitioners.

General Yang Sen's Wine

General Yang Sen was a Chinese longevity expert who was active during the first half of this century. Although he died in his 90's just short of his publicly declared goal of 100, he travelled widely throughout the Far and Southeast Asia teaching the principles of nourishing life and protecting one's health. Below is General Yang Sen's personal formula for a long life wine or tincture. It is given here as an example of a typical traditional Chinese longevity formula. It supplements the *qi*, blood, *yin*, and *yang*. It should not be used by anyone who is not already *yang* deficient. Commonly, this means not before 60 years of age unless otherwise professionally prescribed.

Cornu Cervi (*Lu Rong*), 150g
Colla Cornu Cervi (*Lu Jiao Jiao*), 150g
Colla Plastri Testudinis (*Gui Jiao*), 150g
Gelatinum Corii Asini (*E Jiao*), 150g
Radix Angelicae Sinensis (*Dang Gui*), 60g
Radix Astragali Membranacei (*Huang Qi*), 80g
Radix Panacis Ginseng (*Ren Shen*), 20g
Fructus Rubi (*Fu Pen Zi*), 20g
Fructus Lycii Chinensis (*Gou Qi Zi*), 60g
Placenta Hominis (*Zi He Che*), 60g
Fructus Ligustri Lucidi (*Nu Zhen Zi*), 60g
Herba Cynomorii Songarici (*Suo Yang*), 60g
Gecko (*Ge Jie*), 1 pair
Hippocampus Kelloggi (*Hai Ma*), 2 pieces

93

These ingredients include human placenta, donkey skin gelatin, tortoise shell gelatin, deer antler gelatin, deer antlers, geckos, seahorses, ginseng, *dang gui*, and raspberries among others. Place these ingredients in a large ceramic vessel and cover with 6 liters of strong liquor, such as brandy or vodka. Seal and allow to tincture for 6 months or more. After 6 months, strain and decant half the tincture. Refill the vessel with another 3 liters of alcohol and steep for another 6 months or more. The second time, pour off all the tincture and use, discarding the dregs. Add honey or sugar to taste. Drink 1-2 ounces before bed each night, more in the winter and less in the summer.[3]

Depending upon one's health and general condition, one can use Chinese herbal medicine either to treat existing conditions or merely to supplement waning qi and blood. For instance, I have controlled my own gum disease for years by regularly taking Chinese herbs in pill form. Since symptoms are a sign of imbalance, these symptoms, even if insignificant from a Western point of view, should be treated. The more in balance a person's system is, the more qi and blood they will manufacture. Once a person reaches 60 years of age, almost everyone can benefit from taking Chinese herbal medicine in pill form or wine form, either on a daily basis or at least during each winter.

[3]   Reid, Daniel P., *Chinese Herbal Medicine*, Shambala, Boston, 1987, p. 163

10.

TREATING ILLNESS EARLY

In the preceding chapters we have discussed a number of ways one can help nourish their life and protect their health. These have included a regular lifestyle, proper diet, exercise, rest and relaxation, sexual moderation, self-massage, *qi gong,* and using Chinese herbal supplements. Following these guidelines, one should achieve a new sense of health and energy. However, people being people, we do sometimes get sick. From the Chinese medical perspective, disease is an imbalance in the flow of our *qi* and blood and in the harmony of *yin* and *yang.* Once one is diseased, this disharmony further impedes the function of the organs and bowels and the organism tends to produce less *qi* and blood and to also, therefore, consume more *jing* essence. In fact, chronic disease is listed as one of the ways that our source *qi* becomes weak and wasted.

Because disease is not only the symptom of imbalance but also perpetuates and accentuates imbalance, it is vitally important that one treat disease as soon as it arises. Further, it is important that one eliminate the cause of the disease and not just palliate its symptoms. Medical treatments can be categorized as either root or branch treatments. Branch treatments only address the symptoms. Root treatments seek the root or cause of the disease. If one mows the lawn, one is only cutting off the leaves of the grass. Because the roots are untouched, one must mow the lawn again next week.

Similarly, if one only treats the branch symptoms of a disease, the disease process itself continues.

Traditional Chinese Medicine excels at providing root treatment. Practitioners of TCM seek to see their patients as a whole. They take into account every aspect of their patients in arriving at their diagnosis. Whereas branch treatment for an eye disease may only concern itself with the eye, TCM treatment for an eye disease takes into account the patient's bodily constitution, age, sex, energy level, sleep, appetite, bodily warmth, mood, facial complexion, digestion and elimination, appetite, perspiration, and any and every other bodily function, sensation, or symptom the patient complains of.

Traditional Chinese Medicine also uses benign therapies with a low potential for doctor-caused disease or side effects. In TCM, the body is seen as an interrelated whole. Therefore, it makes no sense to the TCM practitioner if one symptom or part of the body is made better while another body part is made ill. They are all connected and there is only one person. Thus Chinese herbal medicine, acupuncture, remedial Chinese massage or *tui na*, and remedial Chinese dietary therapy all seek to heal the whole person without causing problems anywhere else. All the modalities of Chinese medicine work by reestablishing harmony and balance to the entire organism.

Sometimes an illness is so painful, acute, or life-threatening that even the Chinese doctor must first relieve the symptoms before addressing the root. Emergencies require emergency medicine. However, except for medical emergencies, it is best to seek treatment that goes to the root of a problem. In addition, it is important to seek treatment at the very first sign of disease. When a disease is just beginning, it can be remedied very easily. After it has become established, it may be more difficult to treat. In Chinese medicine, based as it is on the Doctrine of the Mean, there are established healthy norms for most bodily functions. Thus the Chinese doctor can often correct a disease before other medical practitioners even recognize that a problem exists.

For instance, a patient is asked about their bowel movements. They answer that their bowel movements are just fine. However, when asked further, it turns out that they have a loosish bowel movement after every meal. Questioned even further, they say that, yes, there are undigested pieces of food in their stools. According to TCM, a person should have one large bowel movement per day. It should be formed but not hard and neither too light or too dark. From the patient's description of their bowel movements above, the TCM practitioner knows that the patient's spleen *qi* is weak. Since the spleen is the root of *qi* and blood production, either the patient is already fatigued or soon will be. If left uncorrected, they will eventually also display cold hands and feet, lack of strength, and will be predisposed to easily catch colds.

Happily, the TCM doctor not only knows this patient's spleen is weak but also how to strengthen it. The patient is counselled to eat only cooked, easily digestible foods, to stay away from chilled, frozen, or raw foods, not to drink too many liquids with meals, and to go for a short walk after eating. Further the patient may either be given acupuncture at certain points known to supplement the spleen *qi* or be given Chinese herbal medicinals to strengthen their spleen and boost their *qi*.

Therefore, those interested in cultivating life and protecting their health should periodically see a TCM practitioner. These may be either acupuncturists, Chinese herbal doctors, or both. Such practitioners can often identify and correct imbalances long before practitioners of other medicines. Further, if one already suffers from a disease, one should seek treatment from a TCM practitioner as soon as possible while the disease is still easily curable and has not done too much damage. Once a disease becomes too far developed, it may be necessary to use such strong and dangerous treatments as surgery, chemotherapy, radiation, and all the other high tech treatments of modern Western medicine. But when a disease is still relatively recent or not too far developed, it makes more sense to seek a safer, more holistic, and more radical treatment in the sense of really getting at the root.

Finding a Qualified Professional Practitioner of TCM

Traditional Chinese Medicine is a professional medicine as opposed to a folk medicine. Its practitioners should have just as long and much training as their modern Western counterparts, albeit in traditional Chinese medical arts and sciences. Training in Western medicine, chiropractic, or naturopathic medicine in no way confers special knowledge or advanced standing in Chinese medicine. Just as one would not hire a plumber to fix their electrical wiring, one should be sure to seek out a trained, professional practitioner of Chinese medicine.

In the United States, Chinese medicine is largely practiced under the heading of acupuncture. There are currently 40 or more acupuncture and Chinese medical schools operating in America today turning out approximately 500 hundred new professional practitioners per year. Acupuncture is now legal in approximately half the states in the Union. Americans interested in availing themselves of the benefits of professionally practiced Traditional Chinese Medicine living in states where acupuncture is legal can find the names of local practitioners under acupuncture in their Yellow Pages.

Inevitably the question is asked, "How do I know which practitioner is good?" In states where there is licensing, one should begin by only considering licensed practitioners. Secondly, the National Commission for the Certification of Acupuncturists holds national board exams in both acupuncture and Chinese herbal medicine. Practitioners who are NCCA certified in acupuncture put the letters Dipl. Ac. after their name. Practitioners who are NCCA certified in Chinese herbal medicine put the letter Dipl. C.H. after their name. Other things to consider are whether or not the practitioner is a member of state or national professional associations. Such associations have membership criteria and also ethical standards their members agree to abide by. In addition, there is the National Academy of Acupuncture and Oriental Medicine. Fellows of this body are chosen based on their training, research, knowledge, and expertise as well as on their contributions to their profession. Fellows of this national academy append the letter FNAAOM to their name.

However, beyond this, word of mouth recommendation is important. There is hardly a better reference than that a friend or acquaintance you know and trust has been treated by a practitioner and thinks enough of them to refer you to them. When calling a prospective practitioner, the patient should feel free to ask where they were trained, are they licensed, are they NCCA certified, how long have they been in practice, and how many other patients with the same condition they have treated and with what success. In addition, one should also ask what modalities the practitioner uses, how many treatments or how long their condition will require, and how much that will cost.

When treated early in their course, Traditional Chinese Medicine can successfully treat most diseases, both acute and chronic, without side effects, at relatively low costs, and by getting to their root. Therefore, those practicing the cultivation of life should seek treatment from a professional practitioner of TCM at the first sign of disease, including colds and flus, intestinal viruses, allergies, digestive complaints, hormonal imbalances, skin diseases, and autoimmune disorders.

11.

CONCLUSION

The very first chapter of the *Nei Jing* opens with the following exchange:

> Huang Di asks, I have heard it said that in ancient time people lived to 100 years of age. Nowadays, we are already worn out at 50 years old. Is this due to changes in circumstances or to the fault of people?
>
> Qi Bo answers, In ancient times, people lived according to the *dao*. They observed the laws of *yin* and *yang*, were sober, and lived regular and simple lives. For this reason, they were healthy in body and spirit and were able to live 100 years. But today, people drink alcohol like water, they seek out every licentious pleasure, and addict themselves to intemperance. Thus they are not able to live more than 50 years.

This dialogue underscores the Chinese belief that most people should be able to live to 100 years of age if they live moderately and by the laws of nature. The fact that length of life is primarily the responsibility of the individual based on their choices of diet and lifestyle is attested to by Gao Lian in his *Zun Sheng Ba Jian (Eight Essays on Abiding by [the Rules of] Life):*

> One's destiny (*i.e.*, length of life) resides within oneself. It

does not reside in heaven. Ignorant behavior results in dying young. Wise behavior results in prolonging (one's life).[1]

Wise behavior means approaching healthy living from a number of points of view. Trusting in only one regime or practice, such as *qi gong* or a healthy diet, is not enough. This is clearly spelled out by Ge Hong:

> In everything pertaining to nurturing life one must learn much and make the essentials one's own; look widely and know how to select. There can be no reliance upon one particular specialty, for there is always the danger that breadwinners will emphasize their personal specialties. That is why those who know recipes for sexual intercourse say that only these recipes can lead to immortality. Those who know breathing procedures claim that only circulation of the breaths can prolong our years. Those knowing methods for bending and stretching say that only calisthenics can exorcise old age. Those knowing herbal prescriptions say that only through the nibbling of medicines can one be free from exhaustion. Failures in the study of the divine process are due to such specializations.[2]

In the chapters above, we have presented an overview of traditional Chinese teachings on health preservation and longevity practices. Qian Long's 14 secrets are only one

---

[1] Quoted by Sun Guang-ren *et al.*, *Health Preservation and Rehabilitation*, Shanghai College of Traditional Chinese Medicine Press, Shanghai, 1988, p. 20

[2] Ge Hong, *Alchemy, Medicine and Religion in the China of A.D. 320: The Nei P'ien of Ko Hung*, trans. & ed. by James R. Ware, MIT Press, Cambridge, MA, 1966, p. 113-114

formula. Leng Qian of the Ming Dynasty in his *Xiu Ling Yao Zhi (Essentials of Repairing Age)* gives 16 "shoulds" for cultivating life. These include rubbing the face, combing the hair, moving the eyes, covering the ears, clicking the teeth, closing the mouth, swallowing the saliva, raising the *qi, i.e.,* the anus, calming the mind, storing the *shen*, keeping the back warm, rubbing the abdomen (after meals), protecting the chest, squeezing the testicles, keeping silent, and dry-brushing the skin. Ge Hong, who lived during the Jin Dynasty (265-420 AD), gave the following list:

> Therefore, the prescription for nurturing life is this: Do not spit for distance (too much breath would be lost). Do not walk too fast. Do not listen too intently. Do not look too long. Do not sit too long. Do not stay in bed until you get too weak. Dress before you get chilled. Lighten your dress before you get overheated. Do not overeat when you have been starving. Eat only to satiety. Do not overdrink when you have been parched. Do not overdrink. Overeating begets congestions, and overdrinking produces accumulations of mucus. Don't overwork or take too much ease. Don't get up too early or too late. Don't perspire. Don't sleep too much. Don't race your carriage or your horse. Don't strain your eyes to see too far. Don't chew your food so long that it gets cold. Don't drink wine when you are going out in the wind. Don't bathe your body and hair too frequently. Don't overextend your will or desires. Don't scheme to achieve something ingenious. Don't seek too much warmth in winter or too much cold in summer. Don't lie without covers under the stars. Don't expose your shoulders when sleeping. Don't undergo severe cold, severe heat, strong winds, or heavy fogs. Don't overemphasize any of the five flavors when eating...[3]

---

[3]   *Ibid.*, p. 223-224

103

There are any number of things one can do in order to improve their health and prolong their life. The important thing is to devise a plan that works for oneself. In doing so, one should keep in mind Ge Hong's advice on taking care of the little things:

> Losses may be compared with the flame of the lamp
> melting the grease; nobody notices what is transpiring until
> suddenly the light dies. Profit is to be compared with the
> sowing and cultivating of plants. Before anyone realizes it,
> the shoots begin to appear. Therefore, when regulating the
> body and nurturing its life, give care to the little things.
> Even a slight profit is not to be considered unimportant
> and left uncultivated, nor is a slight loss to be considered
> harmless and left unblocked. Greatness is always the result
> of an accumulation of little things; a million results from an
> accumulation of ones. If you can appreciate it when it is
> only a promise and perfect it when it becomes evident, you
> are close to knowing the divine process.[4]

All this being said, however, there is only so much time in the day, and I do not believe that seeking longevity in and of itself should be one's sole purpose and occupation. No matter how many of the above recommendations one puts into effect in their life, there will inevitably come a day when life departs from this body. That is the one incontrovertible statistic. Everyone eventually gets old, gets sick, and dies.

If one spends all their time and effort in attempting to preserve their youth and prolong their years, they will inevitably be disappointed at the end. Rather, I believe it is important to devote one's life to some other goal. If one's life

---

[4]   *Ibid.*, p. 215

is lived for some greater purpose, then living long and healthily is a means to an end rather than the end itself. What good does it do a person to live till 80 plus years of age if one is miserable or unhappy every day. The gypsies judge how rich a person is by how much money they have spent in their life, not how much money they have when they die. Similarly, life becomes valuable in its living and living always involves an expenditure of *qi* and essence.

The Chinese teachings on health and longevity all are based on moderation, but the lamas in James Hilton's famous novel, *Lost Horizons* also advised that one should be moderate in their use of moderation, and Zorba the Greek reminds us to dance.

INDEX

A

A Brief Introduction to the Science of Breathing 85
activity, physical 15
age spots 88
aging 10, 33, 36, 42, 87, 91
alcohol 21, 34, 36, 37, 45, 46, 94, 101
allergies 38, 100
Anderson, Bob 76
animal "herbs" 89
appetite, loss of 56
Arisal of the Clear 38
arsenic trisulfide 89
autoimmune disorders 100

B

Ba Gua Zhang 79
Bai Hui 67
balancing food in the four seasons 33
Bao Hui 48
bao jian 13
Bao Pu Zi Nei Pian 24, 41
bedroom taxation 48
beef 32-34
bones 10, 31, 48, 61, 87, 84, 70, 74, 75
branch treatments 95
breakfast 28
Buddhism 1, 67
bupleurum 89

C

Cai Ji-tong 54
calories 73
Cao Cao 13
Cao Ting-dong 57
celestial drum 62, 66, 67
central nervous system 67

cerebrospinal fluids 79
Chan Tong Qi 77
Chen Ke-ji 3
Chen Ying-ning 1, 60
Chen Zhi 19
chest, pain in the 86
Chi Kung Meditations 57
chicken 34
chilled drinks 34
Chinese herbal medicine 3, 27, 38, 46-47, 87, 90-94, 96, 99
Chinese martial arts 79, 75
Chong Gui-qin 16
Cohen, Ken 57, 77
cold drinks 33, 34
colds and flus 100
concentration, one-pointed 80
conception vessel 59, 60
conforming with nature 13
Confucianism 1
constitutional type, choosing food based on 32

D

damp turbidity 27
dao of sex 47
dao of yin and yang 41
dao sheng 13
Dao Shu 78
dao yin 59, 61, 65, 68, 84, 85
Daoism 1, 77
Daoist History 78
deafness due to old age 66
death 7, 8, 10, 36, 67
deer antler 90, 94
depression 56, 70
dietary therapy, remedial 37
digestion 21, 25-30, 32, 36, 46, 51, 57, 60, 67, 87, 85, 69, 96

digestive complaints 100
dining practices, good 29
dinner 28
dizziness 44, 56
Doctrine of the Mean 97
dong gong 80
Dong Hao 77
donkey skin gelatin 90, 94
du mai 59
duck 34

E

ears 2, 10, 16, 56, 57, 59, 61, 62, 89, 103
earth 3, 13, 14, 24, 25, 67
eating at regular, fixed times 28
eating for longevity 21
eating the right amount 28
ectomorphic 32
eggs 23, 27, 32, 33, 90
Eight Essays on Abiding by [the Rules of] Life 101
ejaculation 42-46
ejaculation, pacing 43
emergency medicine 96
endomorphic 32
Entering the Gate of Medicine 23, 24
essence 8-10, 14, 21, 24, 31, 33, 35, 36, 42, 43, 45-48, 51-53, 56, 60, 61, 65, 66, 87, 89, 78-80, 85, 95, 105
Essentials of Repairing Age 103
euphorbia 89
exercise, aerobic 71-73
exercise, lack of physical 69
external macrocosm 33
Extra Treatises Based on Investigation & Inquiry 25, 47, 48
eyes, sparkle in 9

F

fall 10, 14, 15, 34, 43, 44, 53, 54
fast walking 72
fats 26
feng shui 17-19
field of elixir 61
finest essence 8, 21, 52
fish 22, 23, 27, 33
Five Animal Frolics 78
five phase theory 34
flavors, five 24, 31, 103
food pyramid 26
foods, cold, raw, or uncooked 33
foods, fatty 32
foods, moistening 32, 35
foods, spicy 35
400 Characters on Qi Gong 78
fresh air 2, 18, 79
frozen treats 34
fruits 22, 24-26, 32-34

G

Gan Zhen-yun 78
Gao Lian 101
gate of life 33, 66
gate to nirvana 62, 67
Ge Hong 24, 41, 102-104
Ge Zhi Yu Lun 24, 25, 47, 48
gecko lizards 90
General Yang Sen's Wine 93
genitalia 10, 46, 47
ginseng 89, 90, 93, 94
governing vessel 59, 60
grain qi 22, 70
grains 22-27
greens, dark, leafy 22
growth 8, 10, 14, 15, 46, 85
gums, bleeding 67

H

hair on the top of the head 10
He Shou Wu 91
headaches 66, 86
hearing, diminished 56
heart 31, 34, 47-49, 57, 67, 69, 72, 73
heaven 3, 13, 14, 24, 44, 68, 102
higher mental faculties 9
Hilton, James 105
homunculus 61
hormonal imbalances 100
Hu Bin 85
Hua Tuo 13, 14, 78, 70
Huai Nan Zi 74
Huang Di 101
humanity 13
humidity, moderate 18

I

impotence 66
Inner Classic 14, 24
inner elixir 67
insomnia 44, 53, 87
internal microcosm 33
intestinal viruses 100
irritability 56, 70

J

Jin Zi Jiu Zhuan Ji 36, 37
Jin Zi-jiu 36, 37
Jin Zi-jiu's Collected Writings 36, 37
jing 8-10, 14, 15, 17, 21, 24, 31, 33,
    42-48, 51, 53, 56, 57, 60, 61, 66, 87,
    77, 78, 80, 69, 95, 101
jing consumption 10
jing, postnatal 8
jing production 10

jing wei 21
jogging 72

K

keeping regular hours 15
kidney *yang* 66
kidney *yin* 67
kidneys 8, 10, 34-36, 42, 44, 46, 60, 62,
    66, 90
killing *qi* 19

L

lamb 32-34
Lao Lao Heng Yan 41, 57
Leng Qian 103
Li Chan 23, 24
Li Dong-yuan 9, 23, 27, 52, 53
Li Hong-bo 16
Li Xue-zhen 16
libido 10
lifestyle, sedentary 69
lifting weights 74
limbs, weakness of the 56
Lin, Anna 91
Ling Shu 14, 31
Liu Qing 44, 48
Liu Xiao-ming 29, 54
Liu Zhao-cun 16
longing, unnecessary 55
Lost Horizons 105
lower *dan tian* 61, 62, 65, 67, 80, 83,
    85
Lu Jiu-zhi 70
lunar nectar 67
lunch 28
lungs 8, 21, 35, 36, 52, 90, 79, 80, 85,
    69, 73

M

Ma Wang Dui 77
macrocosmic orbit 68
martial arts, Chinese 79, 75
marrow, sea of 60
massage, remedial Chinese 96
massage, self 4, 59, 68, 85, 76, 95
maturation 10, 15
meals, taking a short walk after 30
meat 23, 24, 28
medicines, patent 91, 92
meeting of hundreds 67
menopause 45
menstrual bleeding, excessive 45
mental clarity 10, 85
mental functions 10
mental stress 46
mental tranquility 54
mesomorphic 32
microcosmic orbit 59, 68
milk 32, 33
ming men 66
misspelling or misspeaking oneself, frequently 56

N

nap during the day 53
National Academy of Acupuncture and Oriental Medicine 99
National Commission for the Certification of Acupuncturists 99
nausea 56
Nei Jing 14, 15, 24, 31, 69, 101
nervous system, central 67
nian si shi, yin qi si ban 33
nocturia 66
noise 18
noodles 27
North Star 67

O, P

oils 23, 26
overwork 46, 56, 103
patent medicines 91, 92
Perennial Sayings in Gerontology 41, 57
perspiration 96
phlegm/damp type 32
Pi Wei Lun 9, 23, 52, 53
pinellia 89
pipefish 89
placenta, human 90, 94
poke root 89
pollution 18
Polygonum Multiflorum 91
polyuria 66
Porkert, Manfred 74
pregnancy later in life 45
prenatal essence 9
Prince Huai Nan 74
Prince Wen Hui's Cook 38
procreation 42

Q

qi 2-4, 7-10, 13-16, 18, 19, 21-23, 26-37, 42, 45-48, 51-54, 56, 59, 60, 65-68, 87-90, 92-94, 77-80, 84-86, 69-71, 73-76, 95, 97, 101-103, 105
qi and blood 15, 16, 27, 28, 30, 31, 33-35, 37, 51, 53, 67, 68, 87, 88, 89, 92, 94, 86, 69, 70, 74-76, 95, 97
Qi Bo 101
qi consumption 10
qi, free flow of 27, 34, 75
qi gong 3, 4, 77-80, 84-86, 71, 76, 95, 102
qi gong, moving 80, 84
qi gong, normal reactions to 85
qi ju you chang 13
qi mechanism 35
qi, original 23, 31

qi production   10
qi stagnation   86
Qian Jin Yi Fang   52
Qian Long   2-4, 13, 30, 35, 59, 87, 81, 102
qing dan diet   22, 23, 26, 38

R

raw *vs.* cooked food   26
reading, lack of comprehension when 56
realgar   89
recreation   42
rejuvenation, physical   42
relaxation tape   57
ren mai   59
ren shen   90, 93
reproductive capacity   10
reproductive essence   42, 46
resistance training   71, 73, 74
rest and relaxation   51
rest, physical   51, 52
rising and dwelling, normalcy in one's 13
Rising Eagle   80
root treatments   95
royal bee jelly   90
rubbing the abdomen after meals   30

S

saliva, swallowing   60
sea of marrow   60
seahorses   89, 94
seal testicles   90
seasons, modifying one's activities to conform to   15
Secret of the Purple Rock   54
Secrets for Keeping One's Youth   78
sedentary lifestyle   69

self-massage   4, 59, 68, 85, 76, 95
semen   42, 43
sex and aging   42
sex without ejaculation   45
sexual abstinence   43
sexual activity, pacing one's   43
sexual vampirism   47
shen   9, 10, 60, 90, 93, 78, 80, 103
shen ming   60
sheng zhi zhi jing   42
shi fan   27
shi yi huan jing   17
shou yi   80
Simple Questions   22, 31, 51
simulacrum   61
skin diseases   100
skin, lustre of   9
sleep   8, 9, 16, 18, 28, 33, 43, 53, 54, 57, 88, 85, 70, 96, 103
sleepiness   56
sleeping habits, good   53
soy sauce   24
Special Treatments for Lung Diseases: Qigong Treatments   77
speech, economy of   4, 52-54
Speer, Dr.   27
spirit   9, 10, 14, 24, 31, 37, 67, 78, 80, 74, 101
spiritual brilliance   60
Spiritual Pivot   31
spiritual transformation   42
spleen   8, 9, 21, 23, 28, 31, 32, 34, 35, 37, 51-53, 56, 60, 67, 90, 69, 97
spring   14, 34, 43, 44, 80
steadiness of thought   9
stomach *qi*   31
stress injuries   73
stretching   3, 4, 69, 71, 74-76, 102
stuffiness below the ribs   86
Su Wen   22, 31, 51
sugars   26
sui hai   60

summer 14, 15, 19, 34, 43, 44, 94, 77, 103
Sun Bing-yan 27
Sun Guang-ren 16, 19, 22-24, 41, 52, 56, 57, 70, 102
Sun Si-miao 16, 19, 22, 23, 38, 47, 52, 57, 71
sunshine 18
Supplements to the Thousand [Pieces of] Gold 52
sweets 26
swimming 72

T

Tai Ji Quan 79
teeth 2, 10, 26, 30, 59, 60, 62, 65-67, 103
teeth, loose 67
tension 55, 66
The Dao of Increasing Longevity and Conserving Life 91
The Encyclopedia of Chinese Medicinals 88
thought and reaction, retardation of 56
Three in One 77
tiger bone 90
tinnitus 16, 44, 66
tortoise shell 89, 94
Traditional Chinese Medicine 4, 16, 22, 23, 27, 38, 41, 52, 87, 70, 96, 98, 100, 102
tranquility, mental 54
transformation 7, 8, 14, 22, 25, 33, 35, 42, 51, 54, 59
treating illness early 95
Treatise on Leisure Diseases 70
Treatise on the Spleen & Stomach 9, 23, 52, 53
tui na 96
turbidity 21, 27, 29, 30, 60, 69

U, V

Understand the Truth 78
United States Department of Agriculture 26
vegetables 22, 25-27, 32-34
ventilation, good 18
vision, blurred 56
visual acuity 10, 87
vitality 3, 9, 89
voice, tone and articulation of 9
vomiting 37, 56

W, X

Wang Zhi-xing 80
water metabolism 35
water rice 27
Wei Bo-yan 77, 78
weights, lifting 74
Western medicine, modern 98
Wine, General Yang Sen's 93
winter 14, 15, 19, 34, 37, 38, 43-45, 90, 94, 103
women and *jing* essence 45
wood/fire type 32
xian xue 1
Xing Yi Quan 79
Xiu Ling Yao Zhi 103
Xu Ling-tai 44

Y

yang 9, 13-16, 18, 19, 23, 25, 32-35, 41, 44, 46-48, 53, 54, 59, 60, 61, 66-68, 87-90, 92, 93, 78, 85, 86, 95, 101
yang qi 14, 15, 18, 33-35, 46-48, 53, 54, 60, 66, 85
yang sheng 13, 88
Yang Si-qin 16
yang vacuity type 32

yang xing 13, 89
yawning 56
Yi Bing Lun 70
Yi Jing 77
Yi Xue Ru Men 23, 24
yin 13, 14, 24, 25, 31-33, 35, 37, 41, 46,
    51, 53, 59, 61, 65, 67, 68, 87, 88, 90,
    92, 93, 84-86, 95, 101
yin vacuity type 32
Yuan Li-ren 29, 54

Z

ze ying zi ran 13
Zhang En-qin 16
Zhang Zi-yang 78
Zhong Yao Da Ci Dian 88
Zhu Dan-xi 24, 25, 47-49
Zhuang Zi 77
zhuo 21
Zorba the Greek 105
Zun Sheng Ba Jian 101

OTHER BOOKS ON CHINESE MEDICINE AVAILABLE FROM BLUE POPPY PRESS

3450 Penrose Place, Suite 110, Boulder, CO 80301

For ordering 1-800-487-9296 PH. 303\447-8372 FAX 303\245-8362

A NEW AMERICAN ACUPUNC-
TURE by Mark Seem, ISBN 0-936185-44-9

ACUPOINT POCKET REFERENCE
ISBN 0-936185-93-7

ACUPUNCTURE AND MOXI-
BUSTION FORMULAS &
TREATMENTS by Cheng Dan-an, trans.
by Wu Ming, ISBN 0-936185-68-6

ACUTE ABDOMINAL SYN-
DROMES: Their Diagnosis &
Treatment by Combined Chinese-
Western Medicine by Alon Marcus,
ISBN 0-936185-31-7

AGING & BLOOD STASIS: A
New Approach to TCM Geriatrics
by Yan De-xin, ISBN 0-936185-63-5

AIDS & ITS TREATMENT
ACCORDING TO
TRADITIONAL CHINESE
MEDICINE by Huang Bing-shan, trans.
by Fu-Di & Bob Flaws, ISBN 0-936185-28-7

BETTER BREAST HEALTH
NATURALLY with CHINESE
MEDICINE by Honora Lee Wolfe & Bob
Flaws ISBN 0-936185-90-2

THE BOOK OF JOOK: Chinese
Medicinal Porridges, An Alterna-
tive to the Typical Western Breakfast by B. Flaws, ISBN0-936185-60-0

CHINESE MEDICAL PALMIS-
TRY: Your Health in Your Hand
by Zong Xiao-fan & Gary Liscum, ISBN 0-
936185-64-3

CHINESE MEDICINAL TEAS:
Simple, Proven, Folk Formulas for
Common Diseases & Promoting
Health by Zong Xiao-fan & Gary Liscum,
ISBN 0-936185-76-7

CHINESE MEDICINAL WINES
& ELIXIRS by Bob Flaws, ISBN 0-
936185-58-9

CHINESE PEDIATRIC MAS-
SAGE THERAPY: A Parent's &
Practitioner's Guide to the Prevention &
Treatment of Childhood Illness by Fan Ya-
li, ISBN 0-936185-54-6

CHINESE SELF-MASSAGE
THERAPY: The Easy Way to
Health by Fan Ya-li ISBN 0-936185-74-0

A COMPENDIUM OF TCM PAT-
TERNS & TREATMENTS by Bob
Flaws & Daniel Finney, ISBN 0-936185-70-8

CURING ARTHRITIS
NATURALLY WITH CHINESE
MEDICINE by Douglas Frank & Bob
Flaws ISBN 0-936185-87-2

CURING DEPRESSION
NATURALLY WITH CHINESE
MEDICINE by Rosa Schnyer & Bob
Flaws ISBN 0-936185-94-5

CURING HAY FEVER
NATURALLY WITH CHINESE
MEDICINE by Bob Flaws, ISBN 0-
936185-91-0

CURING INSOMNIA
NATURALLY WITH CHINESE
MEDICINE by Bob Flaws ISBN 0-
936185-85-6

CURING PMS NATURALLY WITH CHINESE MEDICINE by Bob Flaws ISBN 0-936185-85-6

THE DAO OF INCREASING LONGEVITY AND CONSER-VING ONE'S LIFE by Anna Lin & Bob Flaws, ISBN 0-936185-24-4

THE DIVINE FARMER'S MATERIA MEDICA (*A Translation of the Shen Nong Ben Cao*) by Yang Shou-zhong ISBN 0-936185-96-1

THE DIVINELY RESPONDING CLASSIC: *A Translation of the Shen Ying Jing from Zhen Jiu Da Cheng*, trans. by Yang Shou-zhong & Liu Feng-ting ISBN 0-936185-55-4

DUI YAO: THE ART OF COMBINING CHINESE HERBAL MEDICINALS by Philippe Sionneau ISBN 0-936185-81-3

ENDOMETRIOSIS, INFER-TILITY AND TRADITIONAL CHINESE MEDICINE: A Laywoman's Guide by Bob Flaws ISBN 0-936185-14-7

THE ESSENCE OF LIU FENG-WU'S GYNECOLOGY by Liu Feng-wu, translated by Yang Shou-zhong ISBN 0-936185-88-0

EXTRA TREATISES BASED ON INVESTIGATION & INQUIRY: *A Translation of Zhu Dan-xi's Ge Zhi Yu Lun*, by Yang Shou-zhong & Duan Wu-jin, ISBN 0-936185-53-8

FIRE IN THE VALLEY: TCM Diagnosis & Treatment of Vaginal Diseases ISBN 0-936185-25-2

FLESHING OUT THE BONES: The Importance of Case Histories in Chin. Med. trans. by Chip Chace. ISBN 0-936185-30-9

FU QING-ZHU'S GYNECOLOGY trans. by Yang Shou-zhong and Liu Da-wei, ISBN 0-936185-35-X

FULFILLING THE ESSENCE: A *Handbook of Traditional & Contemporary Treatments for Female Infertility* by Bob Flaws, ISBN 0-936185-48-1

GOLDEN NEEDLE WANG LE-TING: A 20th Century Master's Approach to Acupuncture by Yu Hui-chan and Han Fu-ru, trans. by Shuai Xue-zhong,

A HANDBOOK OF TRADI-TIONAL CHINESE DERMA-TOLOGY by Liang Jian-hui, trans. by Zhang & Flaws, ISBN 0-936185-07-4

A HANDBOOK OF TRADITION-AL CHINESE GYNECOLOGY by Zhejiang College of TCM, trans. by Zhang Ting-liang, ISBN 0-936185-06-6 (4th edit.)

A HANDBOOK OF MENS-TRUAL DISEASES IN CHINESE MEDICINE by Bob Flaws ISBN 0-936185-82-1

A HANDBOOK of TCM PEDIA-TRICS by Bob Flaws, ISBN 0-936185-72-4

A HANDBOOK OF TCM UROL-OGY & MALE SEXUAL DYS-FUNCTION by Anna Lin, OMD, ISBN 0-936185-36-8

THE HEART & ESSENCE OF DAN-XI'S METHODS OF TREATMENT by Xu Dan-xi, trans. by Yang, ISBN 0-926185-49-X

THE HEART TRANSMISSION OF MEDICINE by Liu Yi-ren, trans. by Yang Shou-zhong ISBN 0-936185-83-X

HIGHLIGHTS OF ANCIENT ACUPUNCTURE PRESCRIP-TIONS trans. by Wolfe & Crescenz ISBN 0-936185-23-6

How to Have A HEALTHY PREG-
NANCY, HEALTHY BIRTH with
Chinese Medicine by Honora Lee Wolfe,
ISBN 0-936185-40-6

HOW TO WRITE A TCM HER-
BAL FORMULA: *A Logical Methodology for the Formulation & Administra-
tion of Chinese Herbal Medicine in Decoction* by Bob Flaws, ISBN 0-936185-49-X

IMPERIAL SECRETS OF
HEALTH & LONGEVITY by Bob
Flaws, ISBN 0-936185-51-1

KEEPING YOUR CHILD HEAL-
THY WITH CHINESE MEDI-
CINE by Bob Flaws, ISBN 0-936185-71-6

Li Dong-yuan's TREATISE ON
THE SPLEEN & STOMACH, *A
Translation of the Pi Wei Lun* by Yang
Shou-zhong & Li Jian-yong, ISBN 0-936185-41-4

LOW BACK PAIN: Care & Prevention with Chinese Medicine by
Douglas Frank, ISBN 0-936185-66-X

MASTER HUA'S CLASSIC OF
THE CENTRAL VISCERA by Hua
Tuo, ISBN 0-936185-43-0

THE MEDICAL I CHING: *Oracle
of the Healer Within* by Miki Shima,
OMD, ISBN 0-936185-38-4

MANAGING MENOPAUSE NAT-
URALLY with Chinese Medicine
by Honora Lee Wolfe ISBN 0-936185-98-8

PAO ZHI: Introduction to Process-
ing Chinese Medicinals to Enhance
Their Therapeutic Effect, by Philippe
Sionneau, ISBN 0-936185-62-1

PATH OF PREGNANCY, VOL. I,
Gestational Disorders by Bob Flaws,
ISBN 0-936185-39-2

PATH OF PREGNANCY, Vol. II,
Postpartum Diseases by Bob Flaws.
ISBN 0-936185-42-2

PEDIATRIC BRONCHITIS: Its
Cause, Diagnosis & Treatment Ac-
cording to TCM trans. by Gao Yu-li and
Bob Flaws, ISBN 0-936185-26-0

PRINCE WEN HUI'S COOK:
Chinese Dietary Therapy by Bob
Flaws & Honora Lee Wolfe, ISBN 0-912111-
05-4, $12.95 (Published by Paradigm Press)

THE PULSE CLASSIC: A Translation of the *Mai Jing* by Wang Shu-he,
trans. by Yang Shou-zhong ISBN 0-936185-
75-9

RECENT TCM RESEARCH
FROM CHINA, trans. by Charles Chace
& Bob Flaws, ISBN 0-936185-56-2

THE SECRET OF CHINESE
PULSE DIAGNOSIS by Bob Flaws,
ISBN 0-936185-67-8

SEVENTY ESSENTIAL TCM
FORMULAS FOR BEGINNERS
by Bob Flaws, ISBN 0-936185-59-7

SHAOLIN SECRET FORMULAS
for Treatment of External Injuries,
by De Chan, ISBN 0-936185-08-2

STATEMENTS OF FACT IN
TRADITIONAL CHINESE
MEDICINE by Bob Flaws, ISBN 0-
936185-52-X,

STICKING TO THE POINT 1: A
Rational Methodology for the Step
by Step Formulation & Adminis-
tration of an Acupuncture Treatment by Bob Flaws ISBN 0-936185-17-1

STICKING TO THE POINT 2: A
Study of Acupuncture & Moxibus-
tion Formulas and Strategies by
Bob Flaws ISBN 0-936185-97-X